Adamantine Strength: A Sensible Guide to Strength, Muscle Growth, and Performance

By Andrew J. Obergfell, CSCS

First Edition: May 2019

ISBN: 9781099070006

WARNING

Part 1: Introduction

Chapter 1: Why I Wrote This Book

The thesis of this book is that everyone can benefit from properly-programmed strength training. Lifters and athletes in any discipline can benefit greatly from learning and perfecting certain fundamental barbell movements, creating a logical and sensible progression in training the main lifts, and then, in the same way, layering on supporting supplemental and accessory movements. By adhering to this method, a lifter can make continuous progress from the very first day of training to potentially elite levels, limited only by his or her ambition and perseverance. This thesis perhaps seems fundamental, but if you walk into almost any gym in America, you would see that it is rarely adhered to.

The greatest strength and muscle gains occur through continuous progression on four bedrock movements: the barbell back squat, the deadlift, the bench press, and the strict overhead press. To succeed, a trainee must master the biomechanics, or technique, of these movements, plan to continuously progress on each movement through proper programming, and finally use supporting exercises to raise general physical preparedness, increase muscle size and recovery, and attack weak portions of the main lifts. These principles are relevant to everyone, from the ordinary gym-goer to the seasoned iron warrior, from a high school athlete's first day in the gym to a professional athlete competing at the highest level. The issue is that very few people actually adhere to these principles, and the result is stagnation or injury. Due to a combination of poor biomechanics, poor programming and lack of ascertainable progress, many people interested in reaching their goals quit, athletes get injured, or they simply lack the motivation to carry on. Many times, the individual untethered to any long-term goal will vacillate from one well-marketed fitness brand to another every time the buzz wears off, never really receiving any meaningful satisfaction with their training. Worse yet, many turn to drugs and expensive dietary supplements in an attempt to patch up otherwise poor training principles. Gains made in this way are at best temporal, and at worst destructive to the athlete. Lack of motivation stems from the inability to see progress toward an ascertainable goal. By creating a program where you can see continuous and systematic progress, your motivation will increase, and you will want to continue.

This book is not about giving you a 16-week program or a 10-week program or even a specific "program" as that term has come to be understood. This is designed to be a "teach a man how to fish" book. In short, this book attempts to start you on the road of being your own best coach. It seeks to teach you how to manipulate the proper variables so you can organize your own training in an efficient manner.

The truth is, while there seems to be an increasing number of "camps," so to speak, or designations in the fitness world (*e.g.*, bodybuilding, powerlifting, Crossfit, etc.), there is a fundamental formula underlying each of these disciplines, which, if mastered, will lead you down the path of success in any discipline you choose. All this by way of saying that before you can break a world record in powerlifting or become Mr. Olympia, or a strongman competitor, or become a superior athlete, you have to learn to properly squat 135. This book posits that the reason people fail to make meaningful progress is because they have not laid an adequate foundation to maximize the potential benefits of their training program. Before I was able to put the ideas that comprise this book together, I wasted years of my life doing things that were absolutely meaningless. With this book, I am seeking to save you from that.

When I was younger, no one had even a clue how to develop athletes physically, how to program or how to perform the movements in a safe, efficient manner. Unfortunately, from what

I've seen, many people still don't. Noticing this lack in the industry, I became obsessed with piecing together the methodologies and principles that work, drawing from a variety of sources. After much research and trial and error, I finally found a system that works (this is coming from someone who wasted years doing movements and workouts that were absolutely meaningless). Using the system laid out in this book, I've increased my lifts exponentially. But one thing to note. This is not an exercise science book, or a book on abstract theory. More so, this book is all about application, about practically organizing your training. My main goal in this book is to assist trainees of all types, anyone who wants to make progress in the weight room, by compiling in one place an effective, complete methodology for training.

Before I get started outlining the book for you in greater detail, I would like to introduce myself. To start, I am nothing special. I was never considered the smartest or the best athlete, no one ever looked at me with any real promise or expectation when I was a child. I do not consider myself particularly smart or talented. Where I do believe I excel, however, is tremendous work ethic and the ability to identify patterns and principles. I graduated college at the top of my class and was senior captain of my college baseball team the year we became conference champions. I then went to law school while also starting my career in powerlifting. I earned my law degree and also became a Certified Strength and Conditioning Specialist. When I was not in the court room, I was training young athletes preparing to play sports at the college level. Applying the principles I lay out in this book, these athletes increased in both muscle mass and strength. Now, I practice law full time in New York City, and I realized that the principles I learned in the weight room can be mastered by anyone, lawyer or lifter. If I can, I would like to make it easier for you than it was for me to learn and apply them. I am confident that if I have been able to grasp and apply these principles with some degree of success, you can do the same, if not more.

The following is a roadmap as to how the book will proceed. Part I is the introduction. The first substantive chapter, with the incendiary title, "Admit You Suck," was a chapter I was contemplating leaving out originally, until it occurred to me that it's probably the most important chapter in the book. The number one thing that we must do to get anywhere is put our egos aside. Today, the biggest problem I see is that people are either delusional or so arrogant that they can't possibly get better. Admit that you are weak to get strong. If you can't do this, then there is a strong chance you will not reach your potential. I'll share with you when I finally realized that I sucked, and I'll tell you how that was one of the most important things that's ever happened to me. Next, we will talk about creating a logical structure to build your training upon, namely the training variables we will concern ourselves with, and how your training should be structured. We need to define what our goals are, and we need to organize our training to meet those goals.

Part II of the book is entitled Adamantine Strength, in which we will apply the general principles we discussed in the preceding chapters. We will take it step-by-step, starting with the building blocks, namely the main, core exercises themselves. I will explain how to perform each specific exercise, which is absolutely crucial. If you can't perform the exercises correctly, you are building a house of cards. After that, I will cover how to organize your workouts from your first day in the gym to potentially elite levels. Training is not an *ad hoc* endeavor. It requires you to learn how to organize your training for long-term success. This book is about increasing performance and building strength in a continuous, systematic manner. As in all things, we must start simply and build up complexity as we go. Many times, we see programs in isolation, not understanding that programs are like puzzle pieces, certain methods become more useful at certain points in your training career. You wouldn't take advanced calculus before you learned how to add and subtract. Each has its time and place. What's significant, however, is that good programs all manipulate the same variables, as we will see later. Thus, Part II of this book will help you organize your workouts from your first day in the gym to higher levels of training.

Part III will focus on nutrition and fueling the body for success in the weight room. I will also discuss supplements. Part IV will focus on the mindset and principles required to be successful in the weight room. As Tim Grover wrote in his book entitled *Relentless: From Good to Great to Unstoppable*, you must train the mind to train the body. That said, let's get started.

Chapter 2: Admit You Suck

Socrates once said that, "I know that I am intelligent, because I know that I know nothing." A couple thousand years later, Mark Bell said that it's amazing how much progress you can make when you admit that you suck. The reason I love these quotes so much is because they exemplify what I consider to be the critical flaw that prevents people from being strong, and that is an unwarranted, inflated ego. Instead of really admitting that we don't have all the answers (or even any answers), we create a delusional fantasy that if we can see our top four abs (maybe) under a fluorescent light in the bathroom, then we can convince the Facebook community that we are in shape. In short, the delusion shields us mentally from our weaknesses, inhibiting forward progress. It's easier to create a fantasy than to put in the work. How do I know this is true? Because I spent the first few years of my training life seeing what I wanted to see, not what I needed to see. I thought I knew what I was doing, I had abs and I thought I was strong because I pulled 405, but in reality, I was skinny and weak. The reps weren't quality, it was a mirage.

I'll never forget the day that it all changed. I was on the train going to law school, and I cracked open Jim Wendler's original "5/3/1" book. In a matter of minutes, I was exposed. I felt like Wendler was talking directly to me, essentially he said strip away all the crap and ask yourself a series of simple questions, can you squat, bench, and deadlift? Can you condition? His point was well taken. The reality is that if you aren't strong and you aren't conditioned, you aren't going anywhere. You can jump through all the agility ladders that you want and do all the rotator cuff exercises that you want, but the truth is if you can't establish a base of strength and conditioning, you don't have a shot as an athlete. At that point, I admitted, finally, that I sucked. That has made all the difference.

From there, I decided I wasn't going to be weak anymore. I started the next day with a 185-pound squat to a high box because at the time my hips and hamstrings were so bad that I didn't have a shot of getting to depth. But by the end of that workout, on the last, all out set, I actually, probably for the first time, got a huge pump in my quads. I knew from there that I'd be okay. It would still take years to perfect, and I'm still improving my craft every day, but I am finally on the right path. The moral of the story is that it took me years of spinning my wheels to finally confront myself and say, "hey, you are weak, do something about it." Do not let this be you.

What is unfortunate is that many times, we are the ones holding ourselves back. We create strongholds in our minds that prevent us from moving forward. At some point, if we are lucky, the delusion breaks, and everything falls into place. The point is that it's more than just giving someone a program to do or a series of exercises to perform. A person must actually commit. It's a mental shift that paves the way for the physical shift. In an instant, your thoughts change, and things become more and more deliberate. At this point, people you know will begin to wonder what happened to you. Things you used to be concerned with, like going to bars and T.V. and video games suddenly become less important. Drama at work, gossip, and the general displacement activities that plague our society also become irrelevant and boring to you. These distractions will be replaced with preparing your meals and planning for how you are going to get to the point where you can perform glute ham raises versus bands.

If you don't believe me, take it from God, who instructed the Apostle Paul that "**my power is made perfect in weakness**," leading Paul to conclude paradoxically for the unenlightened reader but quite naturally and logically if you have read this chapter, **"when I am weak, then I am strong."**[1]

Here is the point. Before we can hope to make progress, we must learn to strip away the delusions, strongholds, and roadblocks that plague us daily. We make a decision to live in truth, to be honest with ourselves, to analyze ourselves objectively. Where things are coming up short, we improve them. Where things are lacking, we expose it and make it better. We allow ourselves to chart a path to move forward. If we have to take our deadlift down to 135 and build it back up, we will. If we have to blow up everything and start from scratch, we will. That's what Adamantine Strength is all about. We, like the Apostle Paul, know that when we expose our weaknesses, we pave the way for new strengths to develop. Blessed are the meek, for they shall inherit the earth.

Before we begin, take a minute to really evaluate your training, evaluate your progress. Make a commitment to getting stronger. Make a commitment to learning how to execute the main lifts, even if you have to reduce the weight. Make a commitment to being mentally tough and not making excuses. Make a commitment to be grounded in things that matter and discard things that don't. In short, commit.

---

[1] 2 Corinthians 12: 7-10 (NIV).

Part 2: Adamantine Strength

Chapter 3: 50,000 Feet

I had a tremendous contracts professor in law school. What I took most out of the class was not anything substantive in the law of contracts; rather, it was what she said about her *approach* to conquering law school. She said that in order to understand what was going on you have to learn to look at the material "from 50,000 feet" and fill in the details later. What she meant was that you really need to understand the logical structure first. If you myopically focus on individual facts, you will miss the big picture. Minor facts have no meaning unless they are in context with the overarching structure. The logical structure here is: we must train with a cognizable, steady progression. Many people just try to get as tired as possible in a 45-minute session and call it a day. They do not prioritize performance. The problem with these types of routines is that, while they will make you tired for the day, over time nothing is ever built. To train with steady progression, you need to understand the following basic concepts upon which the program is based.

Concept No. 1: The Goal is to Increase the Main Lifts

There are four main lifts: the squat, the bench press, the deadlift, and the overhead press. These are multi-joint movements that will deliver the most significant strength and muscle gain. These lifts are not unique. They are a staple in any successful program. Our primary focus in designing our training is increasing the main lifts. Everything we do in and out of the gym is focused on this goal; it is the bedrock upon which every subsequent training decision is made. If something we are doing does not contribute to that goal, we cut it out.

There are several reasons why these four main lifts are the central focus:

1) Each are full-body exercises, they require the athlete to stabilize the entire body. Also, larger amounts of muscle are used as multiple joints are involved in moving the load. As a result, more muscle fibers will be activated.

2) These exercises are "infinitely loadable" meaning that we can, in theory, load the exercise a little heavier each time. A dumbbell can only go so heavy, a machine can only stack so much weight, but a barbell can be loaded to potentially infinite sums.

3) They require a tremendous amount of central nervous system coordination. To execute a barbell lift, the athlete must brace and move a free barbell through space, whereas a machine is on a fixed plane and does not require any real coordination.

4) They are hard to do and require you to invest mentally, emotionally, and physically.

5) Progress can be easily measured in the real world. We may not always know our bodyfat percentage, but we all know what our squat is this year compared to what it was last year. This offers validation and allows the athlete to see the fruits of his or her labor, which has a positive effect on training morale.

6) These lifts represent the bedrock functions that our body is designed to perform: Squatting, hinging/pulling (deadlift), and pressing in multiple planes.

7) They will generate a positive hormonal response.

8) Having a base in strength is a proper foundation for any athlete. In short, having a solid foundation will serve you regardless of what you go on to do. You cannot go wrong with building a base of strength and good technique.

9) They make the rest of life generally easier.

I could list a hundred reasons as to why focusing on the listed barbell exercises is superior. And honestly, any halfway respected publication would say the same thing, namely that the basic, core exercises are far superior to, and take precedence over, smaller isolation exercises. Now, just one final point, I know there are some people out there saying "hey, what about the Olympic lifts? What about sprinting and jumping?" It seems like in the sports training world especially, I see a lot of people and institutions advertising that they base their training off the "Olympic lifts." However, I can assure you that if I went in there and asked one of the athletes to perform a picture perfect squat or picture perfect conventional deadlift, he or she would not be able to do it. I've seen it. And this is exactly the problem. While it sounds good in theory, the

Olympic lifts, namely the snatch and clean and jerk, are complex, technical movements. The snatch requires excellent mobility, strength, and explosion. It requires the lifter to grip the barbell with a wide grip while sinking into a squat with the chest up and the spine neutral. The clean and jerk requires similar skill. I have nothing against the Olympic lifts; they are great. And if you want to be an Olympian, and you are starting this training today, this book will be perfect for you. Why? Because the lifts I've isolated are essentially the building blocks of the Olympic lifts. If I can't conventional deadlift or squat, how in the world can I catch a snatch overhead in a full squat? If I can't strict press/military press, how can I jerk limit weights over my head? I can't. It doesn't make sense. But if you can learn these basic movements and do them well, and develop strength in these movements, you will be well on your way to performing the Olympic lifts.

As to sprinting and jumping, both are useful without question, they are indeed fundamental human movements and requirements. However, a squat properly performed will increase your sprint and will increase your jumping capability. Sprinting and jumping are a matter of an application of force, which can be improved by properly programmed strength training. Now, if you are an elite athlete, obviously serious plyometrics should be part of your program, and as you become more advanced as a trainee, you can begin to implement these methods as you begin to train different capacities. However, I am addressing trainees of all backgrounds and levels. If you are new to training, focusing on these four main lifts will establish a strong base around which other things can be added.

Concept No. 2: How to Increase the Main Lifts

Now that we know the squat, deadlift, bench, and press are the movements we need to improve, the next question becomes how we improve those specific movements. The first way that we improve the main movements is through mastering technique. Technical prowess in the main lifts is the bedrock upon which the entire tower of training will be built. It's the classic Scriptural parable of building on bedrock rather than sand. When you build on sand, a faulty foundation, the structure, no matter how well constructed, is susceptible to implode. When you build on bedrock, the structure can be built both wide and tall, and will never falter.

The second way that we improve the main movements is through use of "supplemental" exercises. A supplemental lift is a barbell exercise that mimics the main movement but is different enough to provide a novel stimulus to the body. For example, a close-grip bench press is a supplemental lift to the bench press because it is a barbell lift that is similar to the bench press but different enough that a novel stimulus is placed on the body. Specifically, by moving the grip in, the triceps will be recruited to a greater degree than a bench press with ordinary grip width. If I have weak triceps, I may use this lift to improve my bench, because greater triceps strength will lead to a greater bench press. As you become more adept at identifying your particular weaknesses in the main lifts, and use proper exercise selection to attack them, your progress will become more continuous.

The third way we improve the main movements is through use of "accessory" movements. The purpose of accessory movements is to train the *muscles* involved in the main movement (accessories will include what are commonly referred to as isolation or bodybuilding-style movements). Notice the distinction, the supplemental lift seeks to train the movement, while the accessory lifts train the muscles involved with the movement. The accessories, then, will have less direct carryover to the main lift, but they provide you with the raw material, namely enhanced musculature, which will allow you to become stronger in the main lifts.

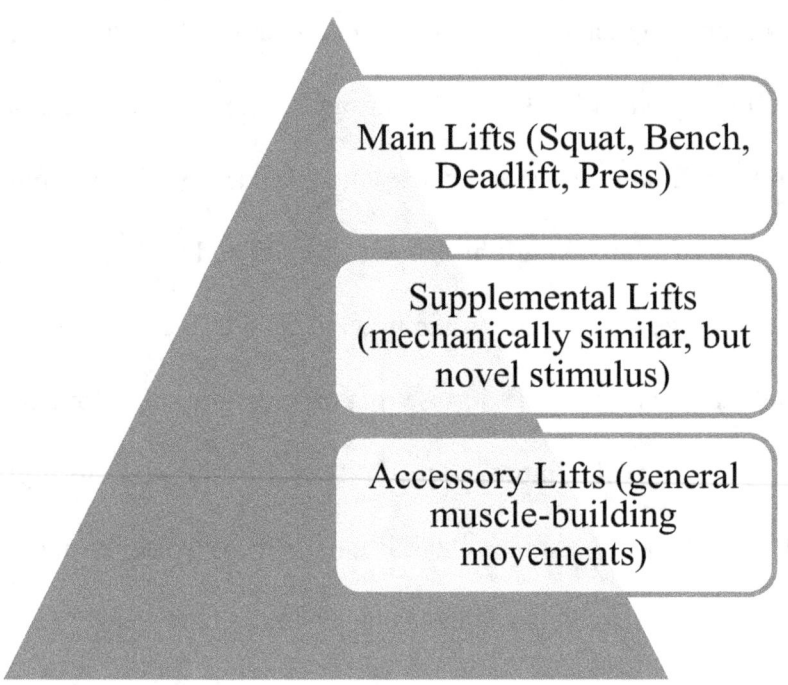

From now on, you will no longer be amused by these arguments and disagreements over whether it is better to be strong or to "feel" the muscle work. You will smirk with wisdom knowing that the answer is both. You will strive to increase strength on the main and supplemental lifts. You will also strive to contract muscle on the accessory movements, knowing that each has its own purpose. This does not mean that the muscles will not be taxed by the main movements. They will. In fact, if you have adequately performed the main lift, you should be perfectly satisfied with your workout if you had to leave the gym at that point. The work on the main lift is the most important part of the workout. However, by properly using secondary exercises, you can continue to fuel progress by attacking weak points in the main lifts, gaining muscle and symmetry, as well as preventing injury.

Concept No. 3: Understanding Volume and Intensity

Programs manipulate two variables that are inversely correlated: intensity and volume. Volume in the exercise science community is defined as the quantity of activity performed in a training session or throughout a training block. For weight training, volume is measured by "volume load," which is calculated by multiplying the sets with the reps with the resistance (volume load = reps x sets x weight used). Intensity is defined as work per unit of time. In layman's terms, volume refers to how *much* work you do, whereas intensity refers to how *hard* the work is done. By way of example, if I perform an absolute maximal effort bench press, intensity is very high (it's the most weight I can possibly push), and volume is very low (one rep). Conversely, if I do a bodybuilding-style dumbbell bench press for 4 sets of 15 reps, volume is very high, but intensity is very low (a far cry from my maximal attempt).

So, you may be asking, what's the big deal? Why does this matter? Well, an effective training program must properly manipulate these two variables. Generally, over the course of a workout, we will start with the highest intensity lift, and taper down to volume work. Working at higher intensities (higher percentages of a one-rep max) is good because it provides a strong neural adaptation, meaning that our nervous system responds to the demand of a heavy lift, becoming more adept at recruiting more muscle fibers than before. Further, higher intensity work requires more mental focus, which is best at the beginning of the workout. Volume, by contrast, provides muscular adaptation, meaning that when we train with more volume, the muscles respond and grow.

Manipulation of volume and intensity is also important over the course of a training block. As we will discuss later, an athlete will want to use volume to increase muscle mass. Then, he or she can gradually shift to higher intensity to train the nervous system to use the acquired muscle to produce a greater force output, resulting in a greater maximal lift. That's why they say that a bigger muscle is a *potentially* stronger muscle, namely because simply adding more muscle mass will not, *ipso facto*, make you stronger. You must include higher intensities to train the requisite neural adaptation to allow for the nervous system to be prepared to move heavy weights. Thus, as you can see, we must concern ourselves with both intensity and volume. Intensity will lead to neural adaptation. Volume will train the muscles and will provide the body with the raw material it needs to perform high-intensity movements.

Chapter 4: Biomechanics: Learning to Execute the Core Movements

I fear not the man who has practiced 10,000 kicks once, but I fear the man who has practiced one kick 10,000 times.

-Bruce Lee

If there is one thing that is absolutely crucial if you are going to be strong, it's that you must master the technique of the core lifts. Until you can learn to master the technique of the main lifts, any strength you build using the wrong way is useless. The idea is to learn perfect execution of the lifts, and then to challenge the technique with increasing loads. If you think of your training as challenging the skill with greater and greater intensities, rather than sacrificing the skill for the sake of greater intensity, you will be well on your way to success. In short, whether you are squatting 135 pounds or 1,000 pounds, it should look the same.

Core Movement 1: The Squat

The squat tends to be one of the hardest movements for most people to learn and perform. Many times, it stems from poor biomechanics. Learning to properly squat requires two things: 1) learning how to adequately breathe and brace; and 2) having sufficient flexibility to execute the lift. The average person starting out will have neither. On the other hand, there are people who are physically capable of squatting correctly but fail to do so because squatting is hard. I can't tell you how many times I've seen a 405-pound quarter squat, and we have all seen the internet videos where some goof loads up the bar and can't descend more than a few inches. This is nothing more than pure ego, which we discussed in Chapter 2. Nothing is less impressive than making a circus of yourself in the weight room. In fact, I have far more respect for the kid who comes in and squats 95 pounds with perfect form. That's the guy that's going to make the real progress down the road.

Now, let's discuss the execution of the squat.

A. Step 1: The Set Up

The setup on the squat is crucial to a successful set. The first thing you must do is set the rack to the proper height, which is usually around your upper chest. You want the bar at a height where you can unrack it with the least amount of energy expenditure. This means not so high that you have to calf raise it out of the rack, but not so low that you are effectively performing a pin squat. We want to save our energy for the movement itself.

When you get the bar to the proper height, then it's time to get organized and get under the bar. First, set your hands. The width of your hand placement will have a lot to do with your shoulder mobility. The key is to set your hands close enough that you can maintain upper-back tightness, but not so close as to cause pain or discomfort. For me, I put my pinky on the rings on a standard power bar. Once you get to a comfortable spot, grab the bar with an overhand grip. My preference is to put my thumb over the bar; I find this is more comfortable. If you want to put your thumb underneath, that is fine also. Once you have your grip, squeeze the bar as if you were bending it into a horseshoe. You will feel your lats engage. At this point, duck your head under the bar and set the bar on a comfortable place on your back (this is usually right on the "shelf" that will be created naturally by your rear delts). Once you are under the bar, think about bending the bar across your back, and you will feel tightness in the lats and upper back. By always thinking of bending the bar across your back, your upper back and lats will remain extremely tight and will prevent you from falling forward during the squat. The lats will also work as spinal stabilizers to keep the back rigid throughout the movement.

Next step is to set your lower half, namely to create external rotation of the hips. To visualize this, think of pushing your knees our as far as possible with your toes pointed forward or slightly angled outward. To help you do this, squeeze your glutes. This will help to center your pelvis under your body.

The last piece before we unrack is to set the ribcage. The way to do this is to simply forcefully exhale, you will feel your abs tighten and pull the ribcage into the proper position. You are now in the power position. Your hips are externally rotated, your pelvis is underneath you and aligned with your ribcage, and your back is tight. This is the biomechanical position in which we can most efficiently apply force. At this point, take a big breath and fill up your trunk with air. In other words, breathe into your stomach. When you establish the proper biomechanical position, it will be impossible to breath anywhere else other than your stomach. If you haven't already, look up such that your head is neutral and in line with the rest of your spine. Now, lift the bar off the rack (keeping your breath) and take two steps back, right foot, left foot. You are then ready to move on to Step 2.

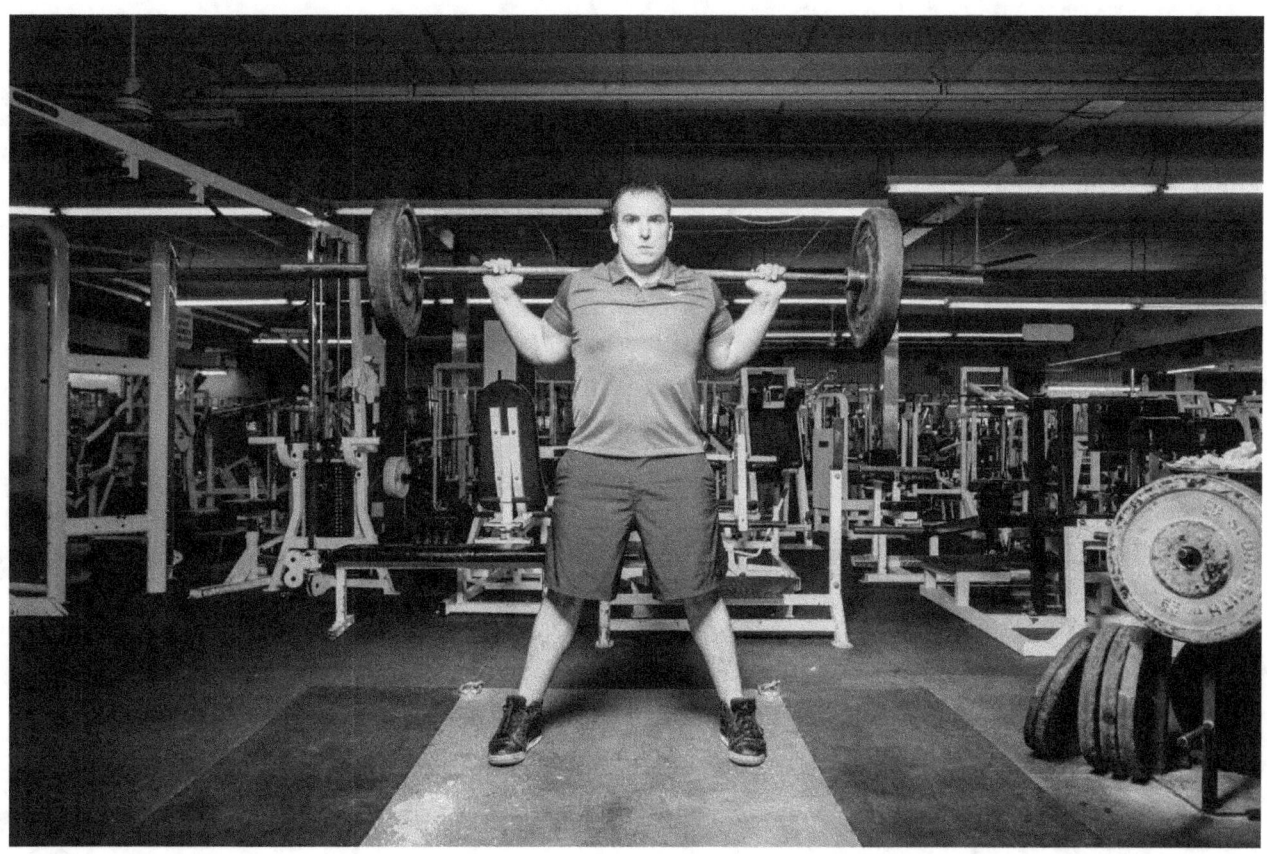

B. Step 2: Maintain Tightness In the Unrack Position

Now that you have the bar out of the rack and are standing with the barbell on your back, all the same principles we discussed during the unrack apply. First, you should be trying to bend the bar across your back—this will keep the upper back tight and help you to stay upright during the squat. Next, you should be squeezing your glutes as hard as possible. With your feet, you should be trying to crack the floor apart between your feet (Note: This does *not* mean that your toes should be pointed out excessively, it only means that you should be seeking to pull the floor apart with your feet. This is a cue designed to stabilize the hips). The idea is to stabilize the hips and to maintain external rotation. From there, pull the ribcage down by flexing and locking the abs down, and get one more deep breath into your stomach. Once you are in this position, you are ready to begin the descent.

C. Step 3: The Descent

Once you get tight in the way I've described above, the rest of the squat is relatively uncomplicated. All I want you to worry about is keeping the glutes tight and forcing your knees out (*i.e.,* maintaining external rotation of the hips to prevent the knees from collapsing inward). Keep bending the bar, which will keep chest up and ensure you do not fall forward. When you reach the bottom of the squat, your knees should be pushed out as far as possible (again, maintaining external rotation), and someone watching you from the front should be able to read the words on your shirt. And as a reminder, you should retain your tightness throughout the descent, meaning you should descend with control and maintain the tightness you created in your back and lower body.

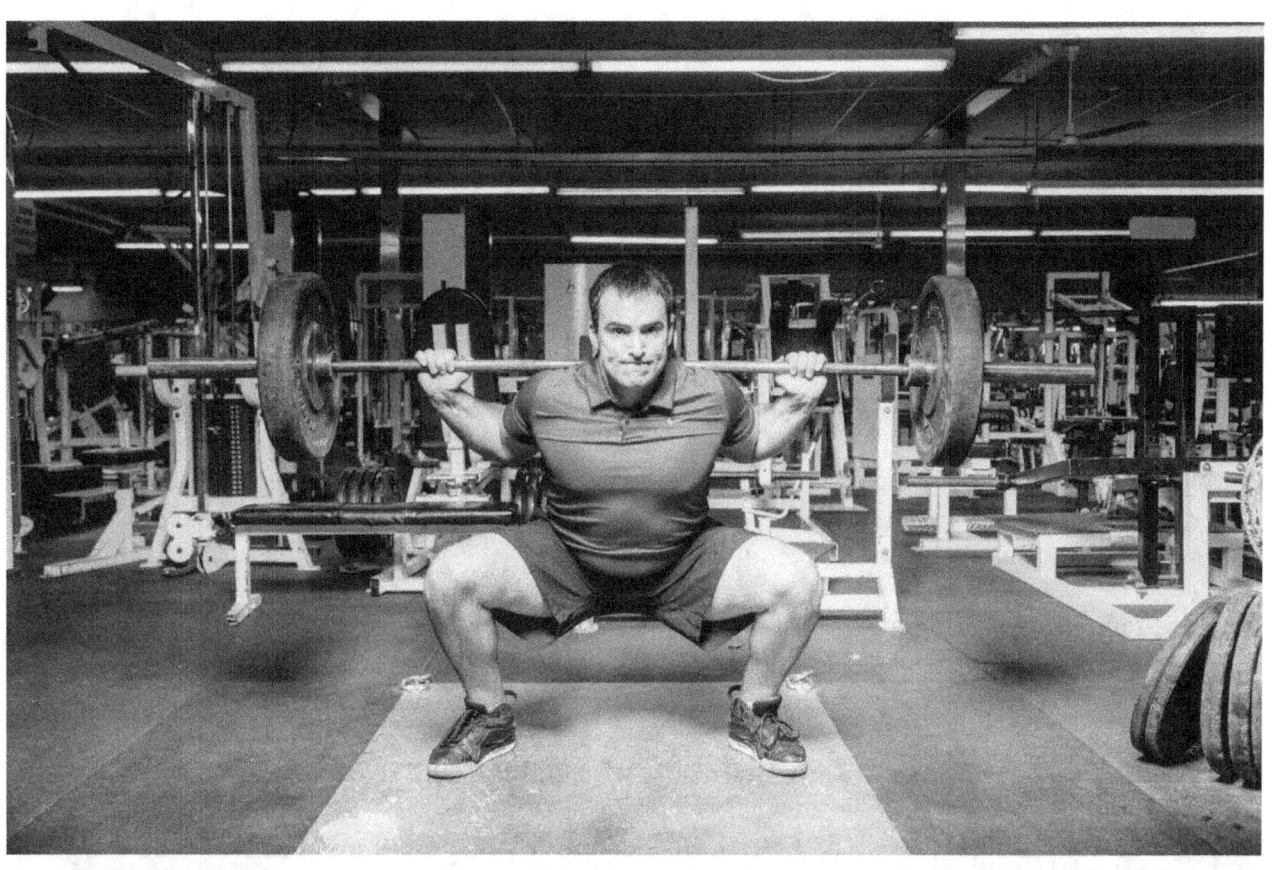

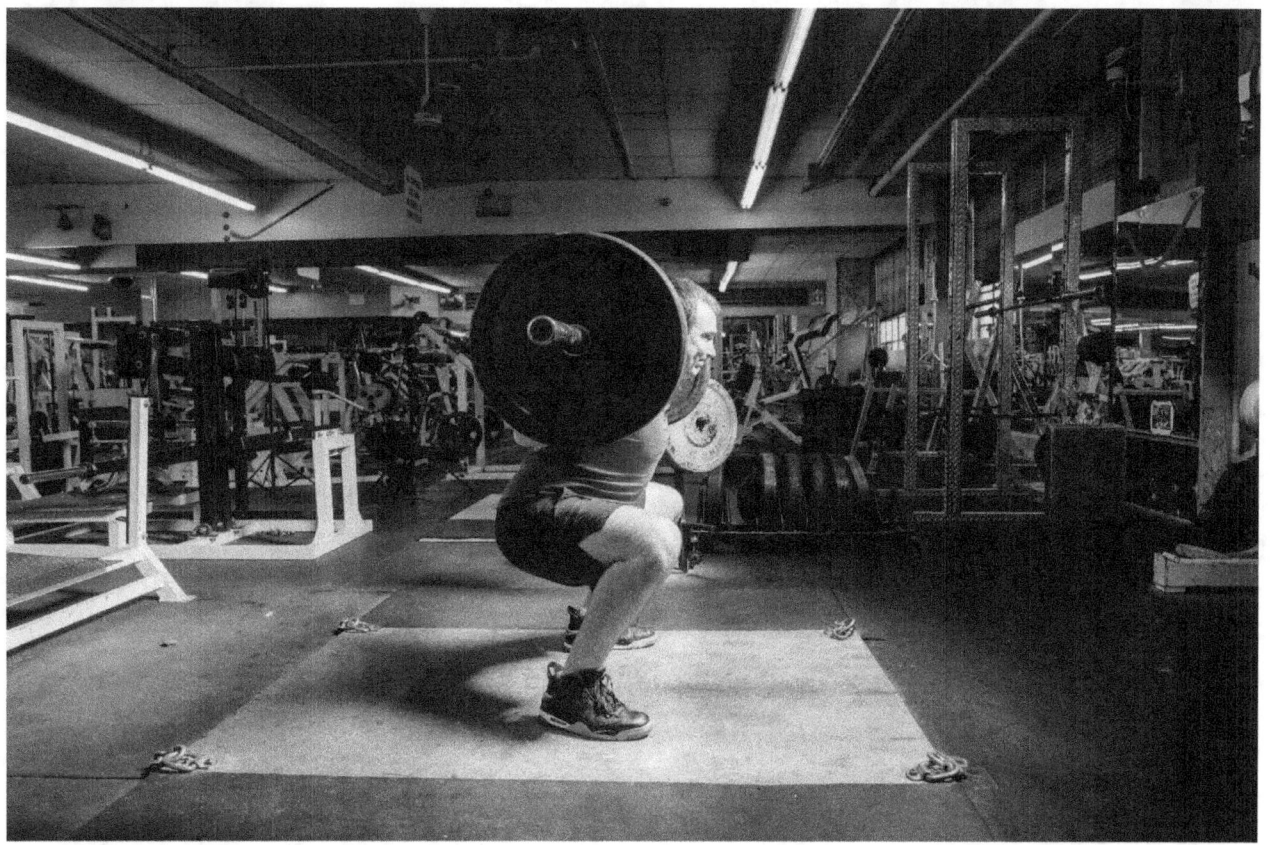

Ordinarily, proper depth for a squat is where the crease of your hips drops below the top of the knee. Depth will have a lot to do with mobility. For most people, if you get the biomechanics right, you can reach depth without a problem. If you are finding that your knees are being pulled in, it likely means your mental focus on generating external rotation of the hips faltered. It could also mean that your groin is very tight, or your hips are weak. If you are finding that your heels are coming off the ground, chances are your hamstrings are very tight. Importantly, your back should remain rigid the entire time. If any part of your back becomes loose or rounds, it is likely due to losing focus on some or all of the biomechanical steps discussed above, but it could also be mobility issues in the chain that are requiring you to compensate by rounding your back. If you are experiencing any of these issues, first check your biomechanics, next check your warm-up (discussed later) to make sure you have sufficiently raised your body temperature to prepare for loaded movement, and third check your mobility.

If you are not hitting depth because your squat will lose 100 pounds, refer to Chapter 2.

D. Step 4: Reversing the Weight

When you have reached proper depth in the hole, you must maintain your tightness. If you get it right, you should feel a "bounce" or stretch reflex from the hamstrings. Importantly, you must keep your knees out at all times, do not let your knees drift in. When you feel this "bounce" out of the hole, continue to forcefully drive the bar up to lockout. When you reach lockout, return to Step 1 and start again. Treat each rep like a single rep to ensure quality throughout the set.

Core Movement 2: The Deadlift

The deadlift is by far my favorite exercise, but it is also the most butchered exercise I see performed. The deadlift requires tremendous focus on stabilization. Otherwise, it will turn into a train wreck very quickly.

There are two types of deadlifts: conventional deadlift and sumo deadlift. Whether you pull sumo or conventional is a matter of body structure and personal preference. You will have to experiment to figure out what variation is best for you. You should train both until you develop a strong preference toward one or the other, and once you do you should continue to train the other as a supplemental lift or a variation on the main movement.

A. Executing the Conventional Deadlift

The conventional deadlift setup will be with a close stance and the hands outside of the legs. As a general rule, your stance should be the same width as if you were going to attempt a maximum vertical jump. The barbell should be over your mid-foot. Many of the same stabilization patters used for the squat will apply to the deadlift. You should be trying to split the floor in half with your feet, and you should be squeezing your glutes.

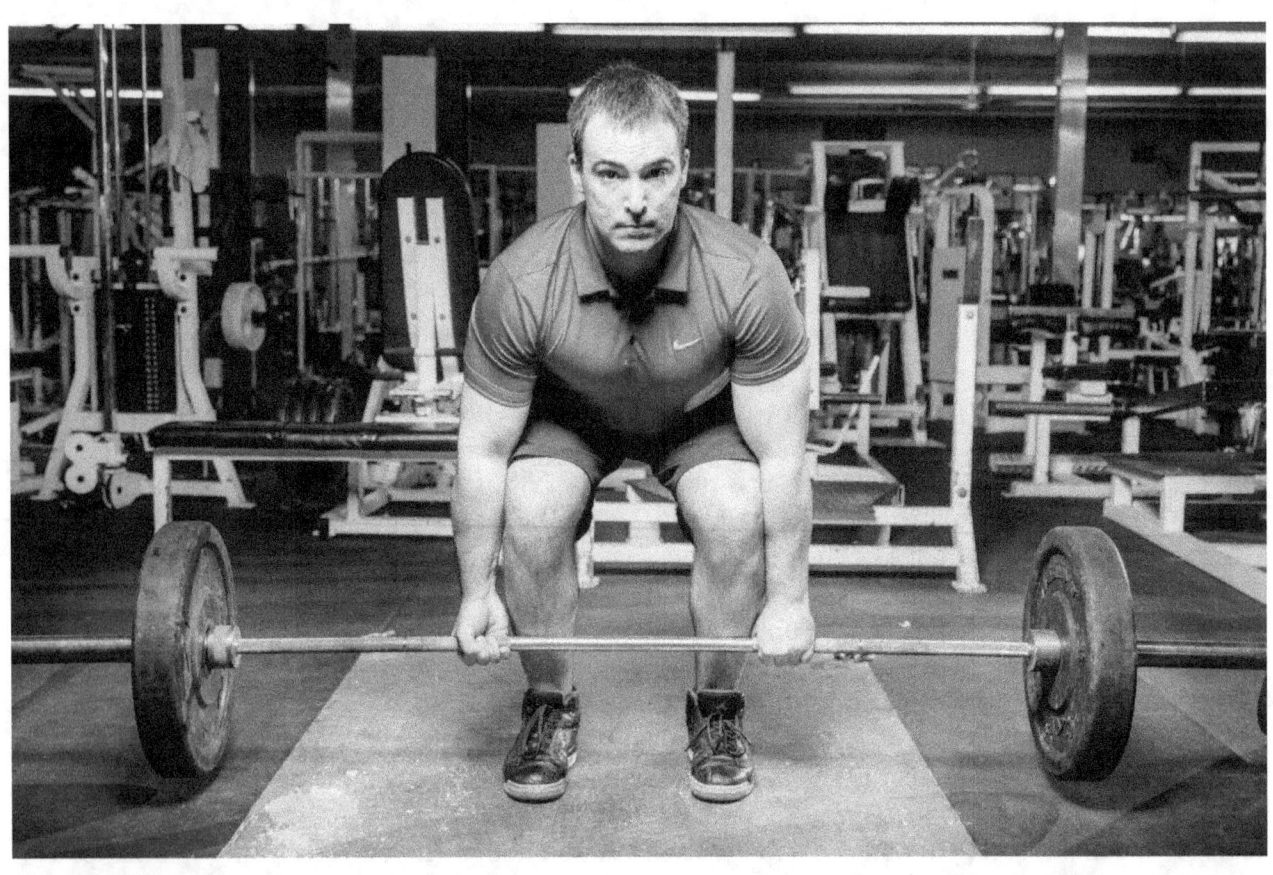

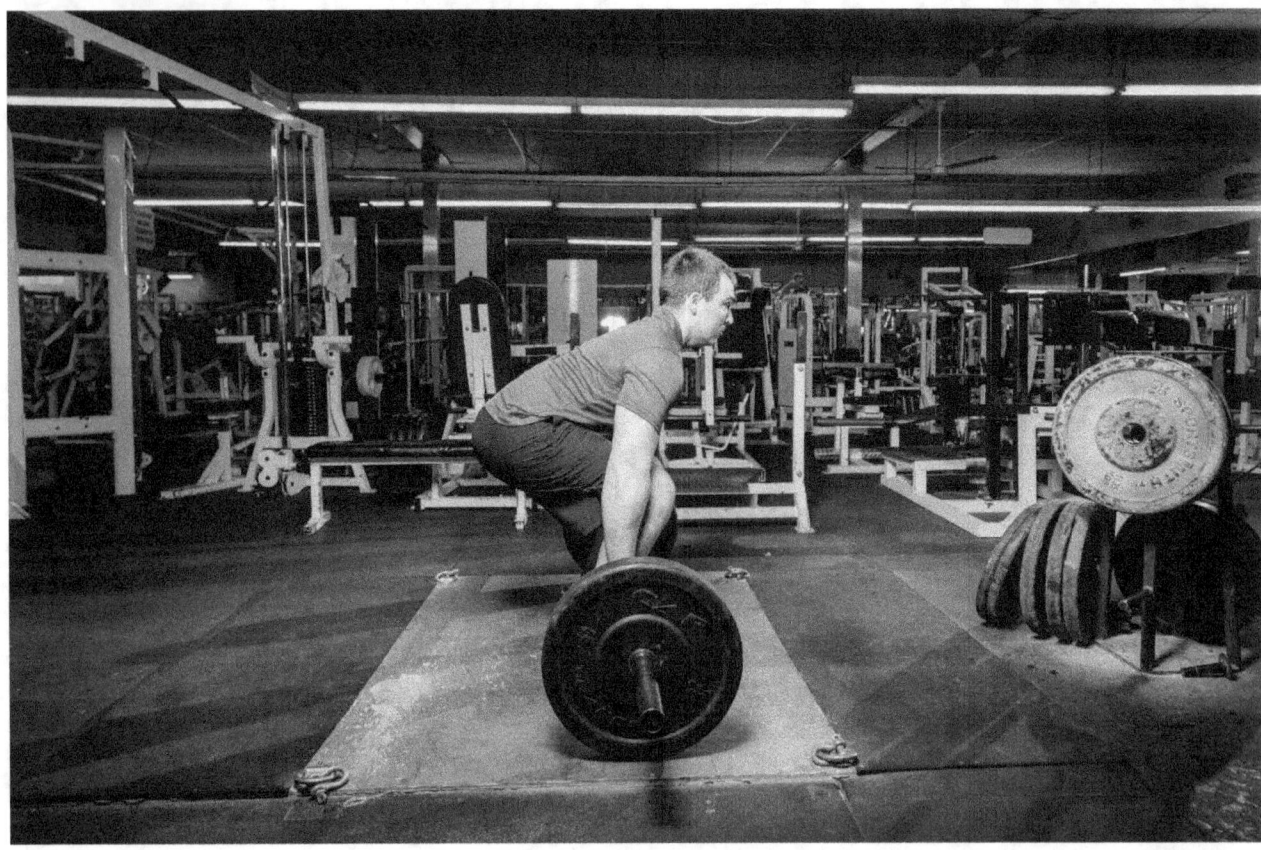

Next, hinge with your hips to activate the hamstrings. A good cue for this is to place your index finger in the crease of your hips, and push them back. You will begin to feel tension in your hamstrings. Now, lower your hands to the bar and grab the bar just outside your shins. When you grip the bar (use a double overhand grip for as long as possible), you should be trying to bend the bar in half. This will engage the lats. This will also result in pulling the "slack" out of the bar. When you have done that, get a deep breath into your stomach. Then, leveraging against the bar, pull your hips down and your chest up, this should bring the bar up against your shins. This position should create a tremendous amount of tension in the system, the bar will want to come up. From there, look up such that your head is neutral with the rest of your spine. You should still be seeking to crack the floor between your feet and get the knees out, as with the squat. Once you have your air and everything is completely tight: *Drive your feet through the floor. Do not "pull" on the bar*.

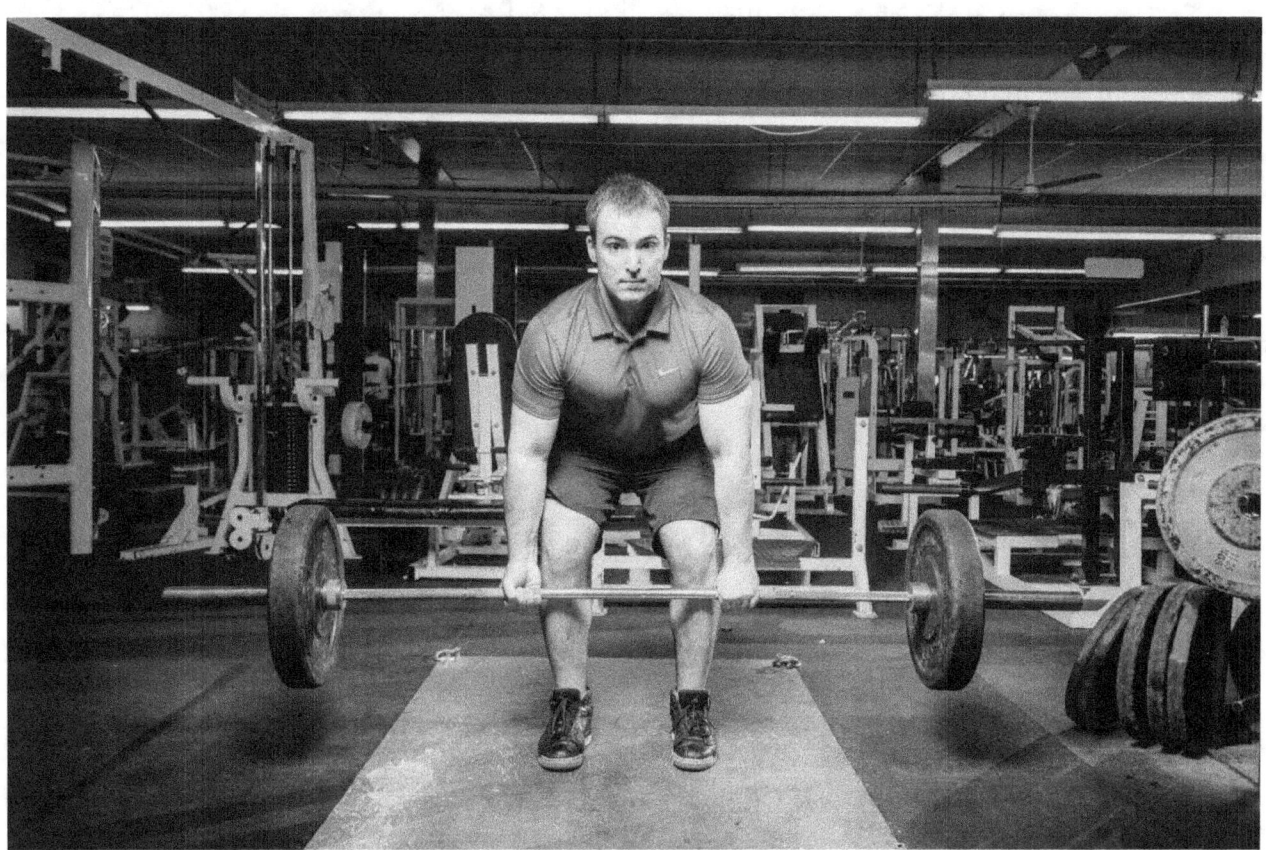

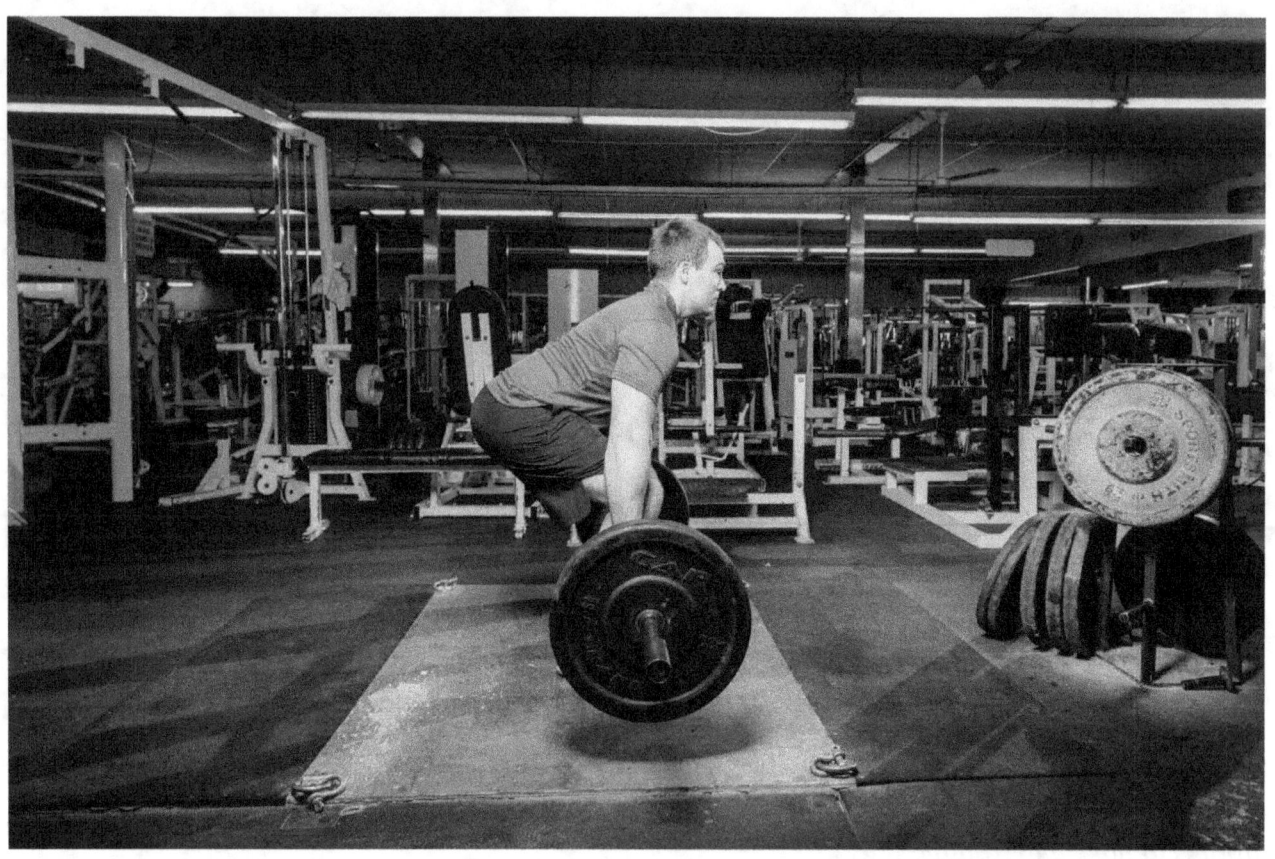

The function of your lats and filling your torso with air is to keep your spine rigid and supported in a neutral position. If, when you start the deadlift, your back immediately defaults into flexion, then you were not tight when you initiated the pull; there is slack somewhere in the system that must be addressed. Until you get this right, **<u>do not</u>**, for any reason, add weight to the bar.

The finished position on the deadlift is when you are standing with your knees locked and your shoulders back. Do not shrug the bar. Do not overextend at lockout. Just think about getting your hips to the bar as quickly and forcefully as possible. You want as little wasted motion as possible. Think tight and fast the entire time.

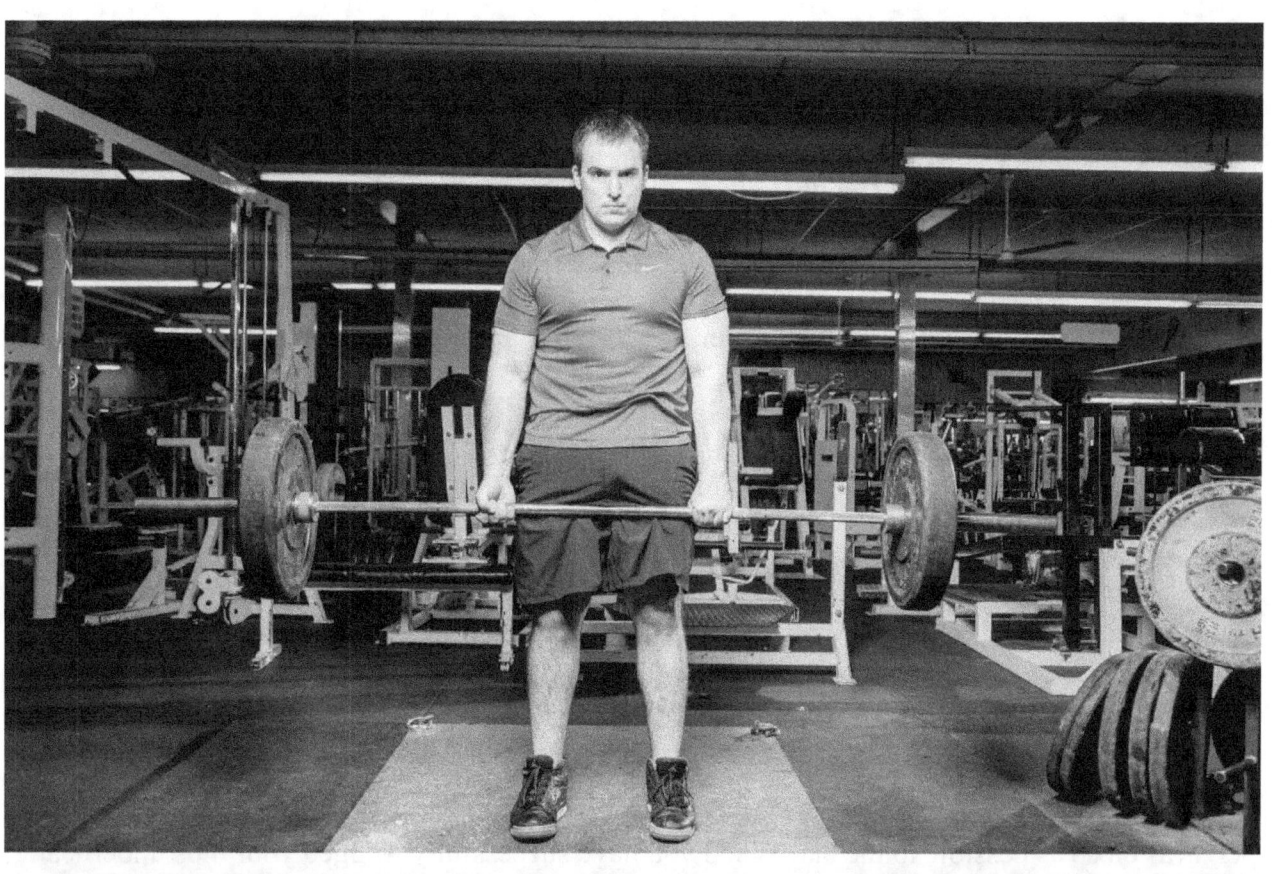

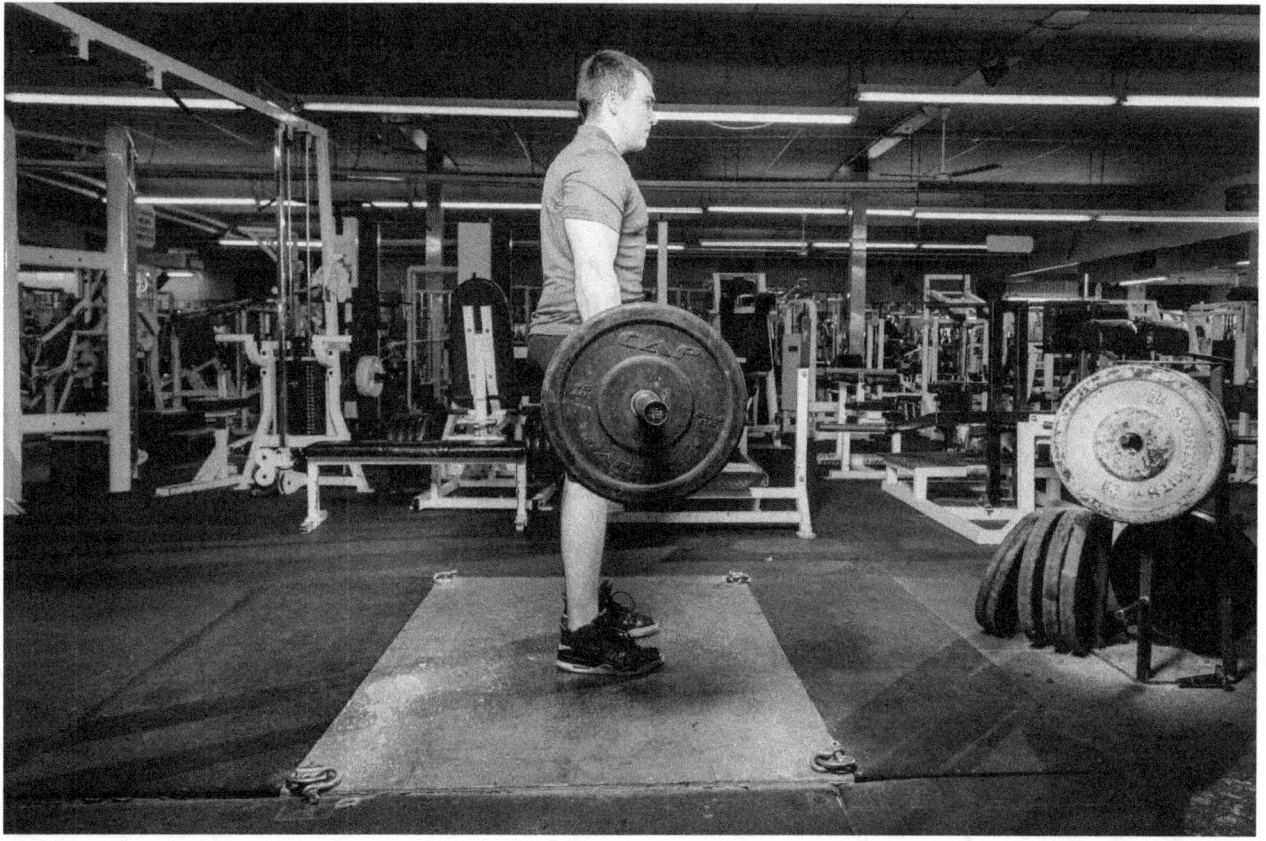

From there, re-establish your starting position and go again. Treat each rep like a single to ensure quality throughout.

B. Executing the Sumo Deadlift

The sumo deadlift is different from the conventional deadlift in that your hands will be inside your legs and your legs will be wider, but the cues and stabilization pattern is largely the same. Unlike the conventional deadlift, you will set up with the bar up against your shins rather than over the mid-foot. The lower-half stabilization pattern, however, is identical. Try to crack the floor between your feet, get the knees out, and squeeze the glutes to pull your pelvis underneath you. Your toes can be rotated out slightly, approximately 15 degrees. From there, force your knees out to descend and grab the bar. Once you grab the bar, stabilize the lats and get a big breath into your stomach, and then leverage your hips down against the bar. Try to get your pelvis as close as possible to the bar. When you have successfully wedged your hips underneath, you should feel the same tremendous tension as the conventional deadlift (the bar should want to come up). Before initiating the lift, look up such that your head is in line with the rest of your spine, and begin the movement.

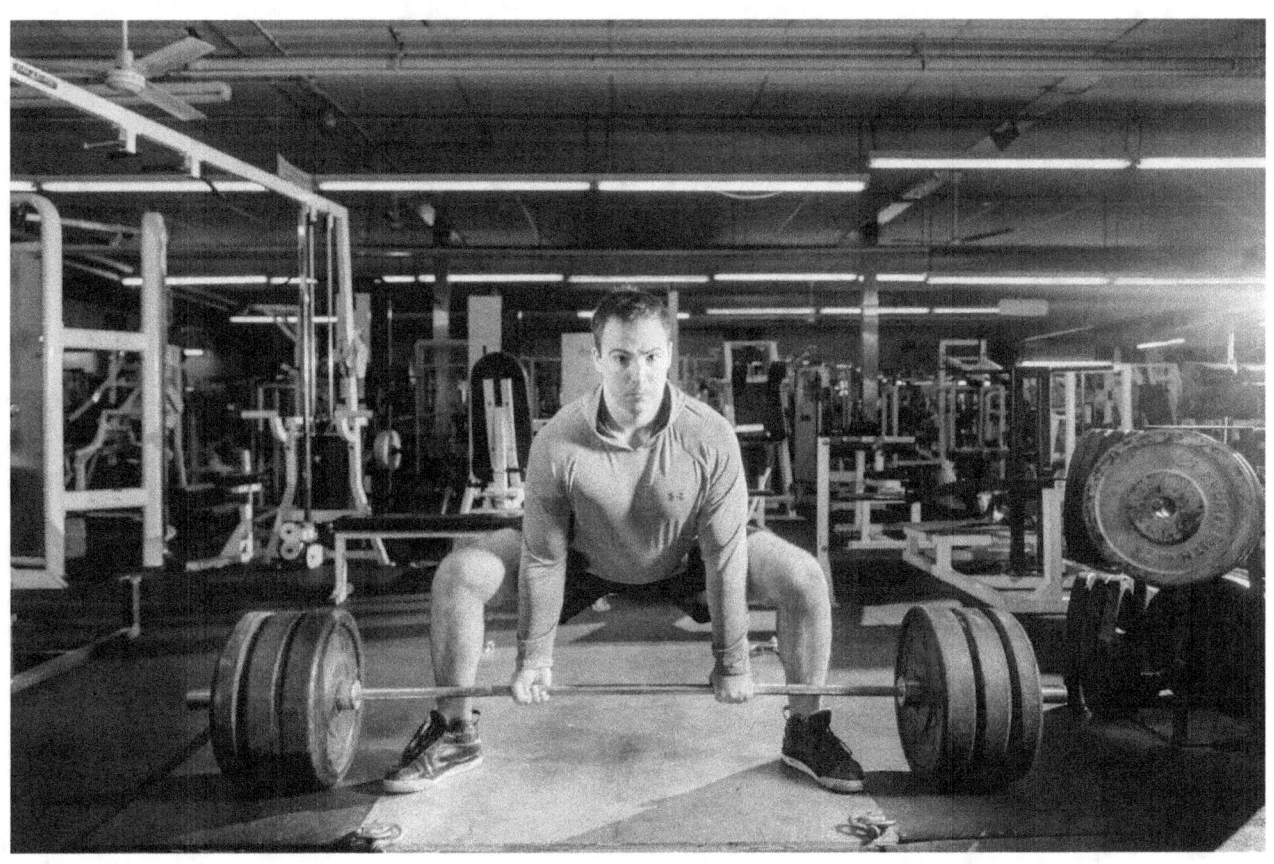

One key tip with the sumo deadlift is to think about forcing your knees out and pulling

back on the bar. Unlike the conventional deadlift, if you think about driving through the floor,

what will tend to happen is that your knees will collapse and come in and you will get pitched

forward. Instead, keep thinking about splitting the floor, and keeping the knees out. Simply pull

back. This will keep you in good position.

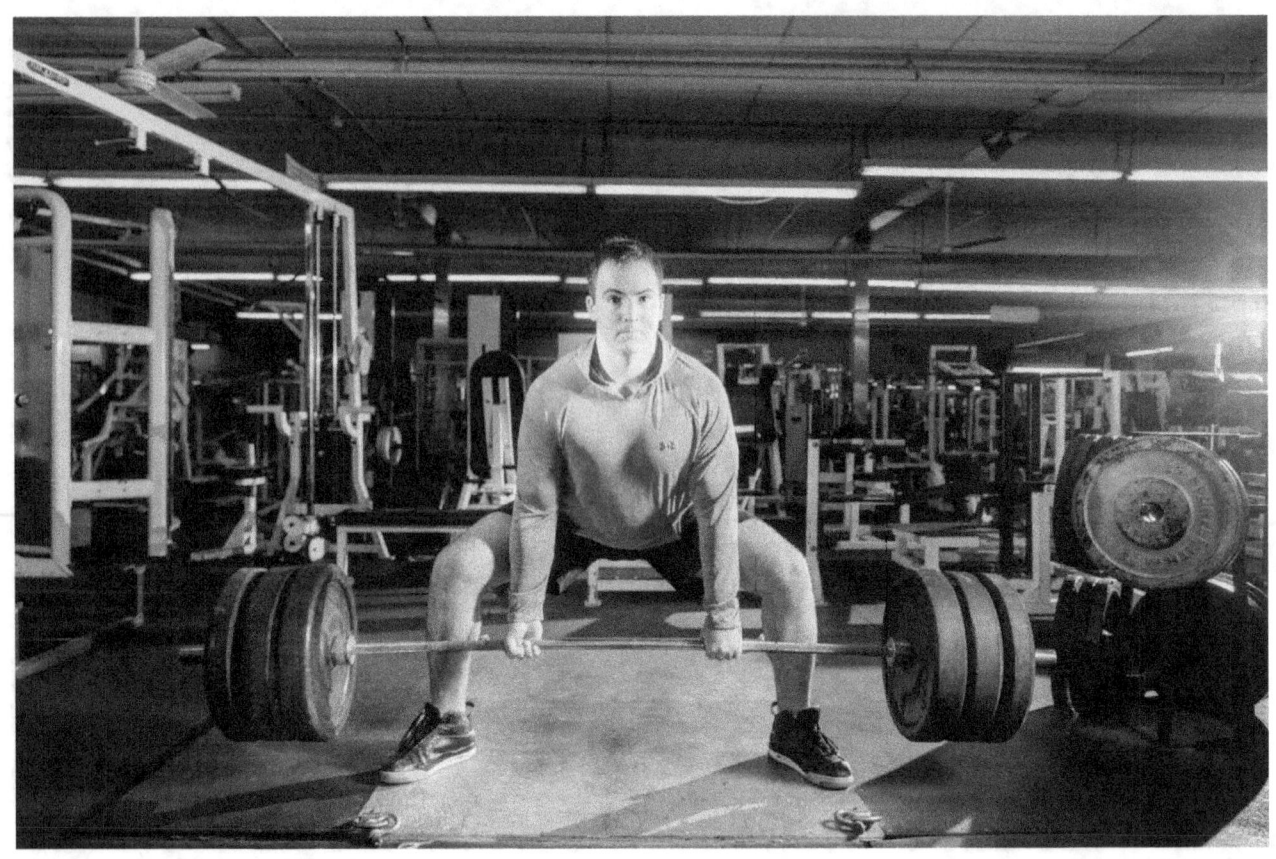

Again, the lockout is as simple as locking your knees at the top with your shoulders pulled back. The load is moved with the quads, hips and hamstrings. Your upper body is just there to stabilize. Do not shrug the bar and do not overextend. Just get the bar to lockout as quickly and efficiently as possible. The deadlift should look crisp and tight. No wasted motion.

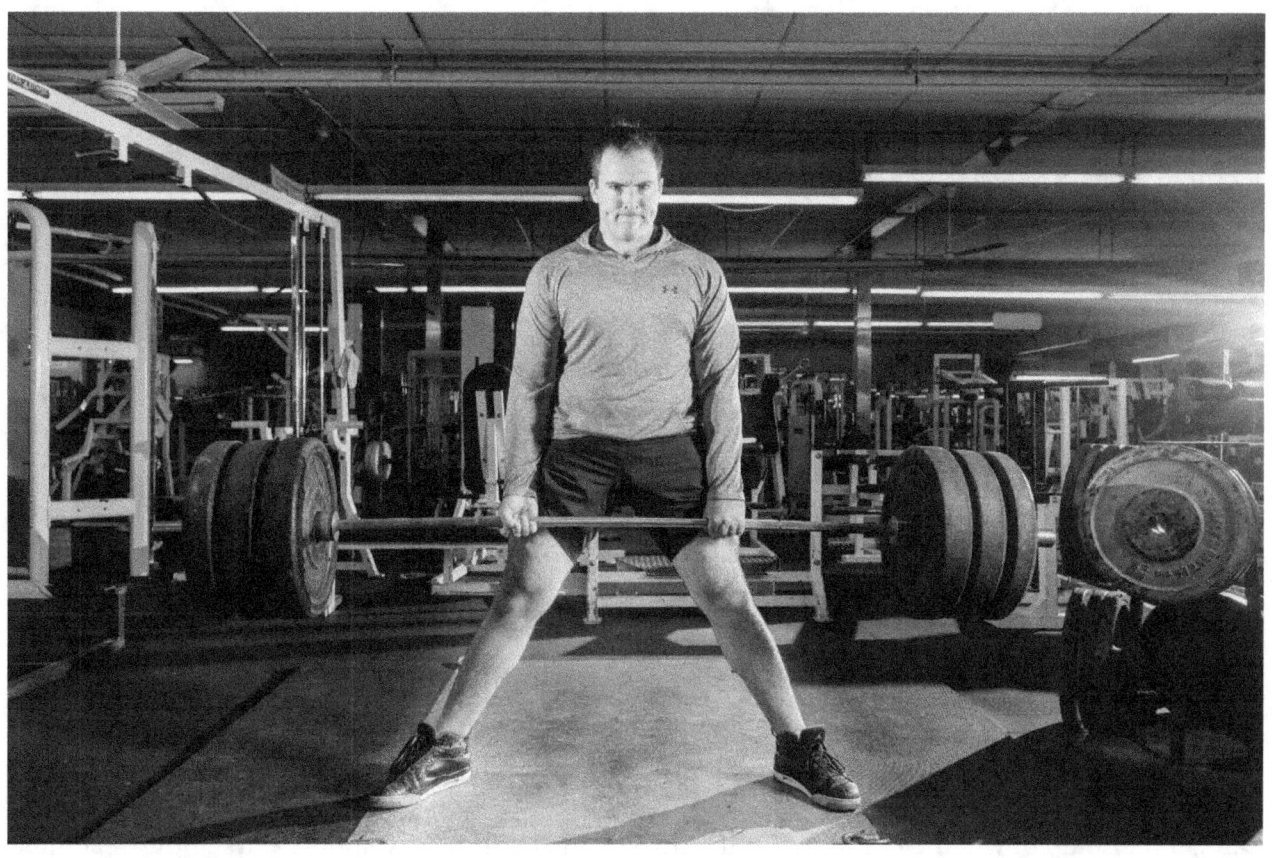

When you have completed the rep, reverse the weight as if you were pressing rewind, and when the bar touches the floor, re-set for rep two. Again, we are looking for perfect technique on every rep, not just performing reps for the sake of performing reps. A final important point about the sumo deadlift is that it tends to feel a little "slower" off of the floor than the conventional deadlift. This is normal when the weights get heavier and you maintain perfect technique throughout. I mention this because some people capsize mentally over this phenomenon. There is no reason to. Simply maintain technique. Be patient in the lift, and know that the bar will pick up speed after a certain point. Fight the temptation to allow yourself to round or be pitched forward. Do not sacrifice technique for the sake of speed.

Core Movement 3: The Bench Press

The bench press is likely the easiest exercise to master because you are lying down and you don't have to worry about quite as many things as with the squat and deadlift. There are three important steps to the bench press. First, you must generate upper back tightness by shifting your weight onto your traps. Second, you must lock the shoulder blades back and down to allow the lats to engage and support the weight. Third, you must generate external rotation with the hips and provide a stabilized base with which to leg drive. When you have the proper setup and execution, you should never have a shoulder or elbow issue from the bench press. If you are finding that your shoulders are getting beat up from the bench, you are losing your tightness and letting your shoulders flare forward. If your elbow hurts, it's because your lats aren't tight and your elbows are flaring out. Now, to make sure we have this right, let's take an in-depth look at the bench press from beginning to end.

A. The Bench Press Setup

The number one problem I see with the bench press is that people just aren't tight. If you can get the setup down, the execution of the lift itself is really pretty simple. First, your feet must be firmly anchored to the floor. I prefer to get a slightly wider base (almost like a sumo deadlift setup), which I find makes me more stable and allows me to generate horizontal leg drive through the barbell. Many times, when the weight gets challenging, people start kicking their feet around violently. That's garbage. I'm not quite sure who ever thought it was a good idea to kick your feet around like a flailing fish while you are trying to press a weight. In any event, the key is this, we must anchor our feet to the floor to provide a strong base. What I want you to do is the following:

1. Lay your feet flat on the floor at your sides.
2. Stabilize sitting on the bench *in the same way you stabilized for the squat and the deadlift*, meaning seek to pull the floor apart with your feet and get the knees out (external rotation).
3. Then, lay back on the bench, your chin should be roughly under the bar.
4. From there, squeeze your shoulder blades back and down (the result should be that your traps are now digging into the bench and your back is slightly arched). You can use the bench apparatus to help you get tight. By this point, you don't want to feel loose

31

anywhere. You should bring your feet as far underneath you as possible and try to pull your shoulder blades into your back pockets. (Note: At this point, you may leave your feet flat on the ground, or if you prefer, drive into the ground with on your toes) This will create tremendous tension on the bench.

5. Then, grip the bar at a comfortable spot. Use the bar as leverage to push your traps into the bench. Then, engage the lats by trying to bend the bar into a horseshoe. At this point, everything should feel tight.

6. Next, pull the bar **straight out of the rack** (Note: Do *not* lift the bar up and out because you will lose your tightness that you just created by squeezing your shoulder blades back and down). As you are pulling the bar out, continue to pull your shoulder blades back and down.

7. Once the bar is over your body at the starting position, continue to try to bend the bar into a horseshoe. At this point, your whole body should be tight.

8. The last step will be to get a large breath into your belly to lock everything down.

9. Once you have done this, you are ready to move on to Step 2, the descent.

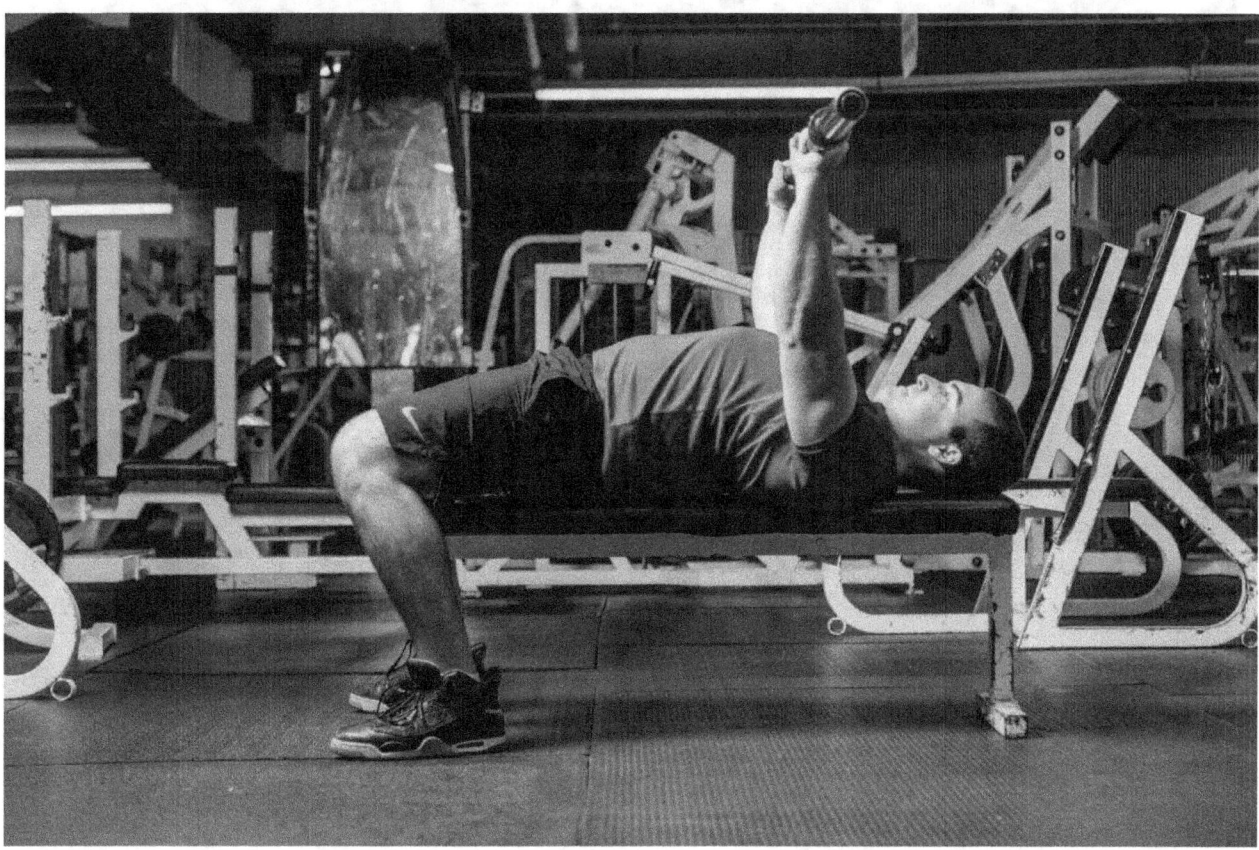

B. The Descent

Once you have effectively completed Steps 1-9 above, that's already more than half the battle. All you have to do from there is stay tight. As you begin the descent, make sure you keep your lats tight. This is most easily accomplished by just continuing to bend the bar on the way

32

down. When you reach the chest, your wrist should be pointed straight (*i.e.,* aligned with the forearm). Thus, your arms should be forming about a 90-degree angle. If your lats are properly engaged, they should resist the descent of the bar and give you an initial push off the chest.

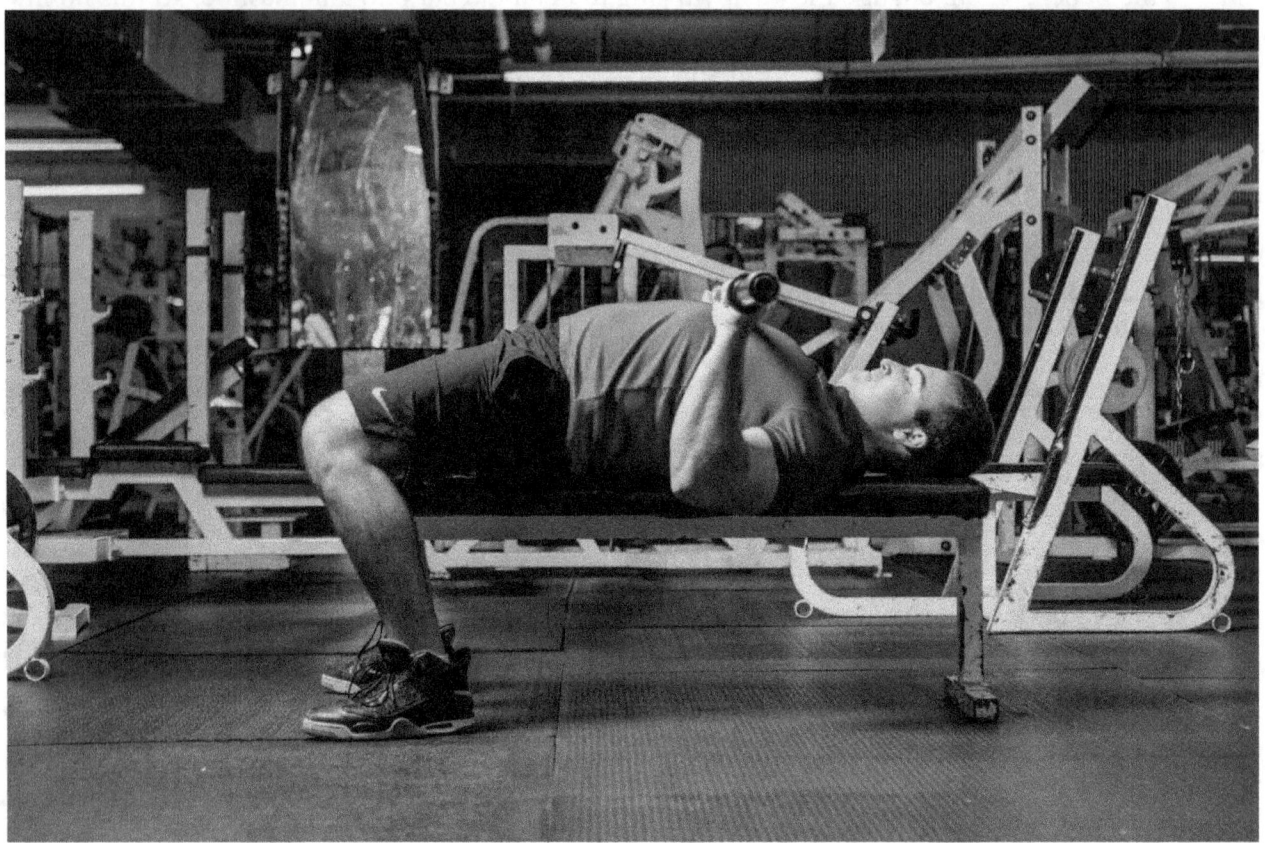

C. The Lockout

When the bar touches the chest, immediately reverse the bar and drive with the legs to get the bar off the chest and drive the bar straight to lockout. Remember, your lower half should be tense throughout the entire movement. When the bar touches the chest, drive with the legs back toward the top of the bench. Think of it this way, when I bench, the bench press will actually move back toward the wall because I'm driving back with my legs. Your butt should not come off the bench. If you have proper tightness, that should not be an issue. People's butts come off the bench because they have not created adequate tension at the beginning of the lift. You should already have maximum tension throughout the system.

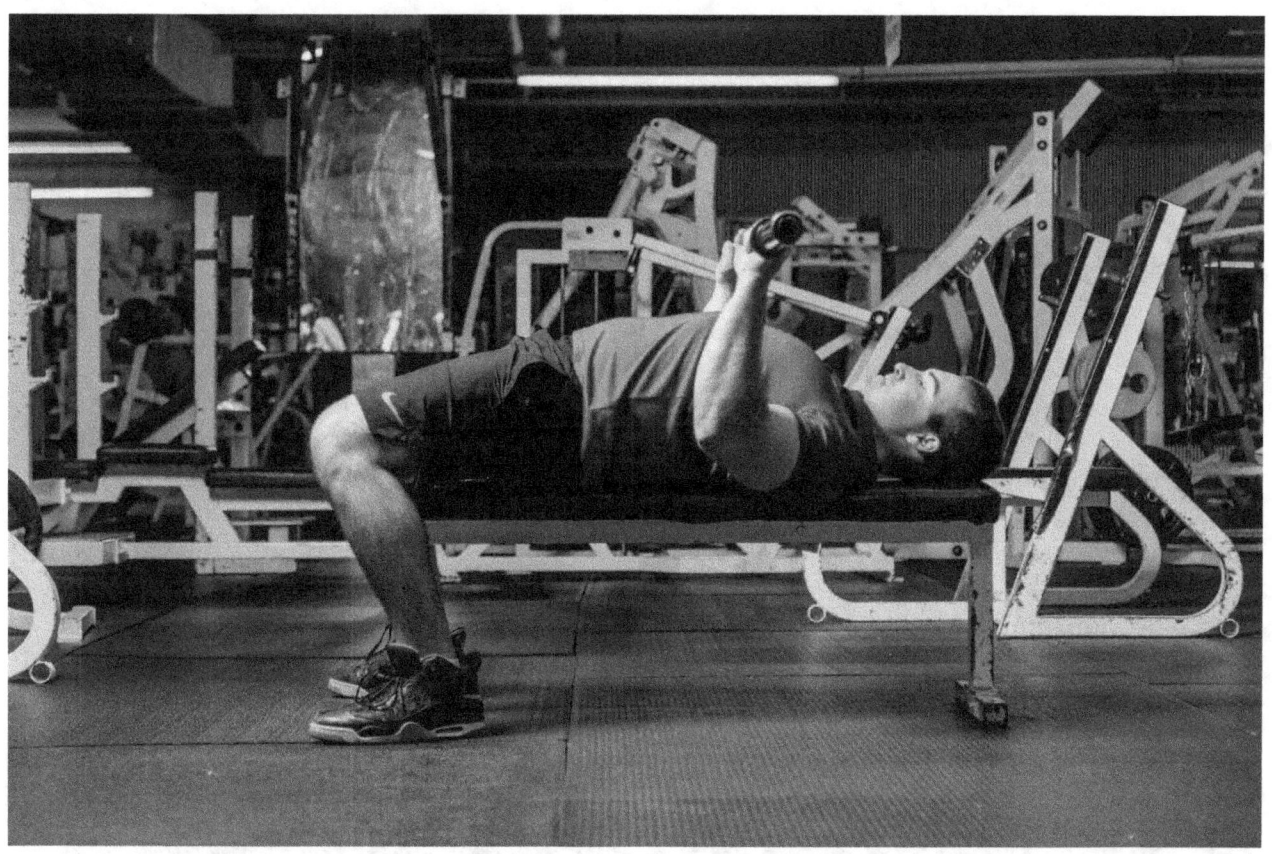

One final thing, as I mentioned before, do not allow your shoulders to roll forward when pressing the weight. This is a recipe for injury. Instead, think of driving yourself back into the bench. Don't think about pushing the bar away from you. If you think about pushing yourself into the bench, your shoulder blades will stay pinched, and you will retain your tightness and shoulder health.

Core Movement 4: The Strict Press

The strict press is a standing, vertical press. To execute the strict press, you must keep the bar close to the center of your body at all times (*i.e.*, imagine a line cutting your body in half). Retract your shoulders back and down and bend the bar in the same way that you do on the bench and squat. Maintain that tension throughout. This keeps the bar closest to your midline and allows you to press with the most strength possible. To execute the press, you must be completely stabilized throughout your whole body.

A. Step 1: Unracking the Bar and Finding Tightness

When executing the military press, the crucial part of the lift is the setup. First, set the bar in a power rack at about the height of the upper chest. What I recommend is to take a grip on the barbell about a thumb's length into the knurling of the bar (assuming a standard power bar). Once you grab the bar, immediately engage the lats by trying to bend it into a horseshoe. From there, duck under the bar, and immediately shelf the bar close to your body. You should be stabilized in the same way as the squat, with the hips externally rotated and glutes tight. You should not have any flexion or extension of the spine. Your body should be straight and vertical. In this position, unrack the bar. From there, take two steps back (left foot, right foot) and proceed to Step 2.

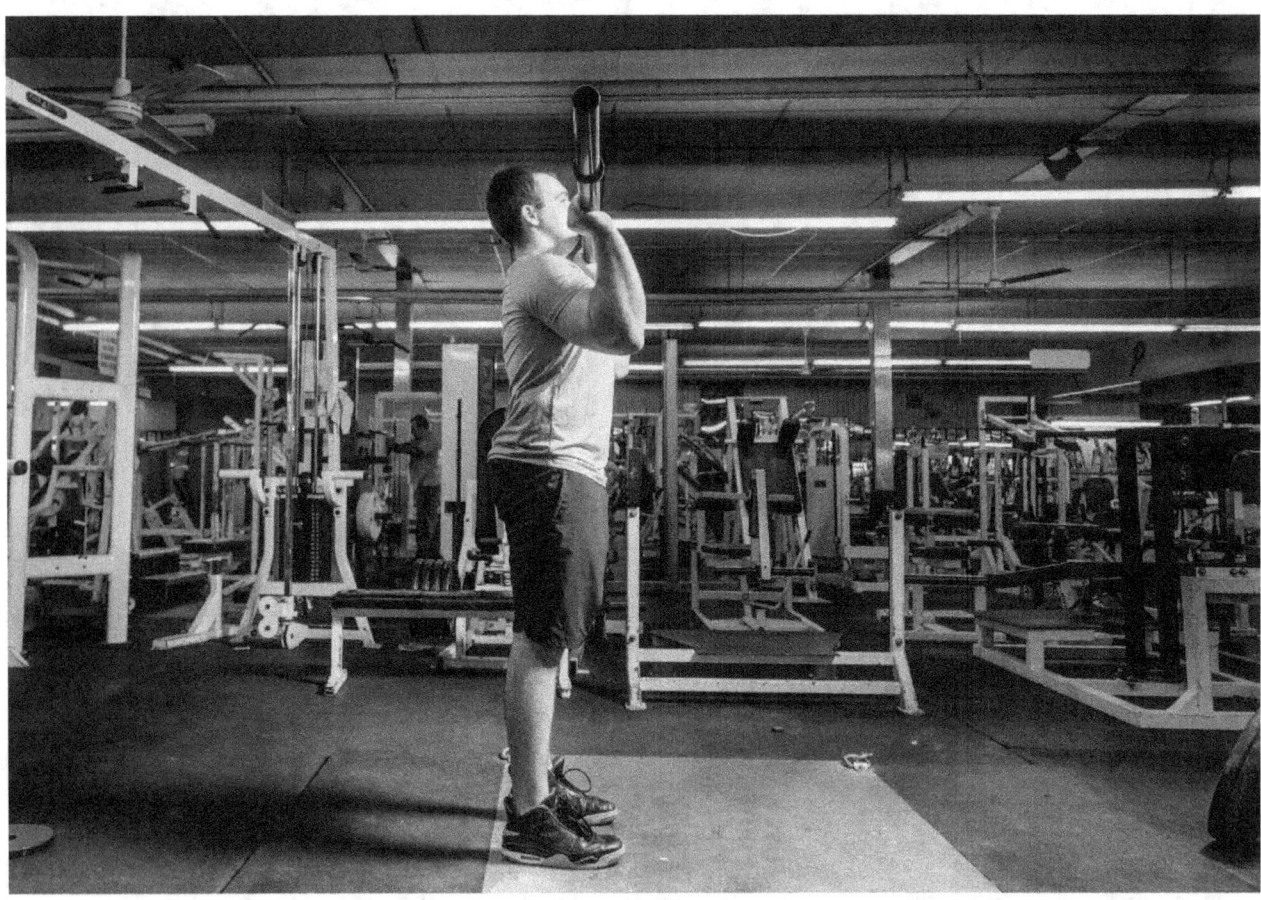

B. Step 2: Stabilization

When you reach the position where you have taken the bar out of the rack, you must generate torque with your feet in the same way you did with all of the lifts mentioned above. (Remember, torque your feet out as if you were trying to split the floor in half between your feet. You should be squeezing the glutes hard.)

As for the upper half, your elbows should be actively pulled in such that they are pointing forward. Do not allow your elbows to flare out. To visualize, think armpits forward. You should feel tremendous tightness throughout your entire body. Finally, keep the ribcage down. This means that your body should look like a straight staff from the side throughout the entire range of motion of the press. You should not hyperextend your lower back (*i.e.*, do not make your body look like a crescent moon). If you are, it could be a mobility issue. More likely, it is just that you are using too much weight.

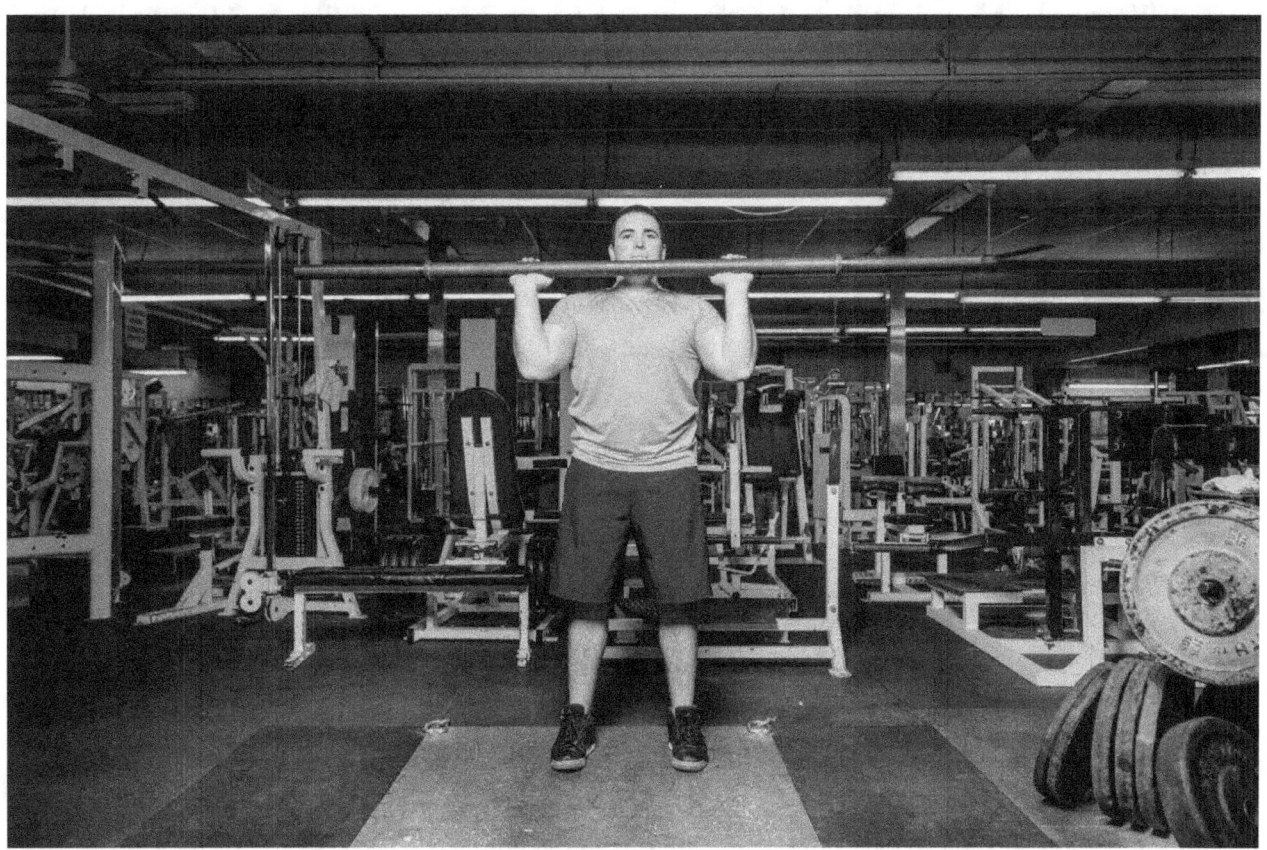

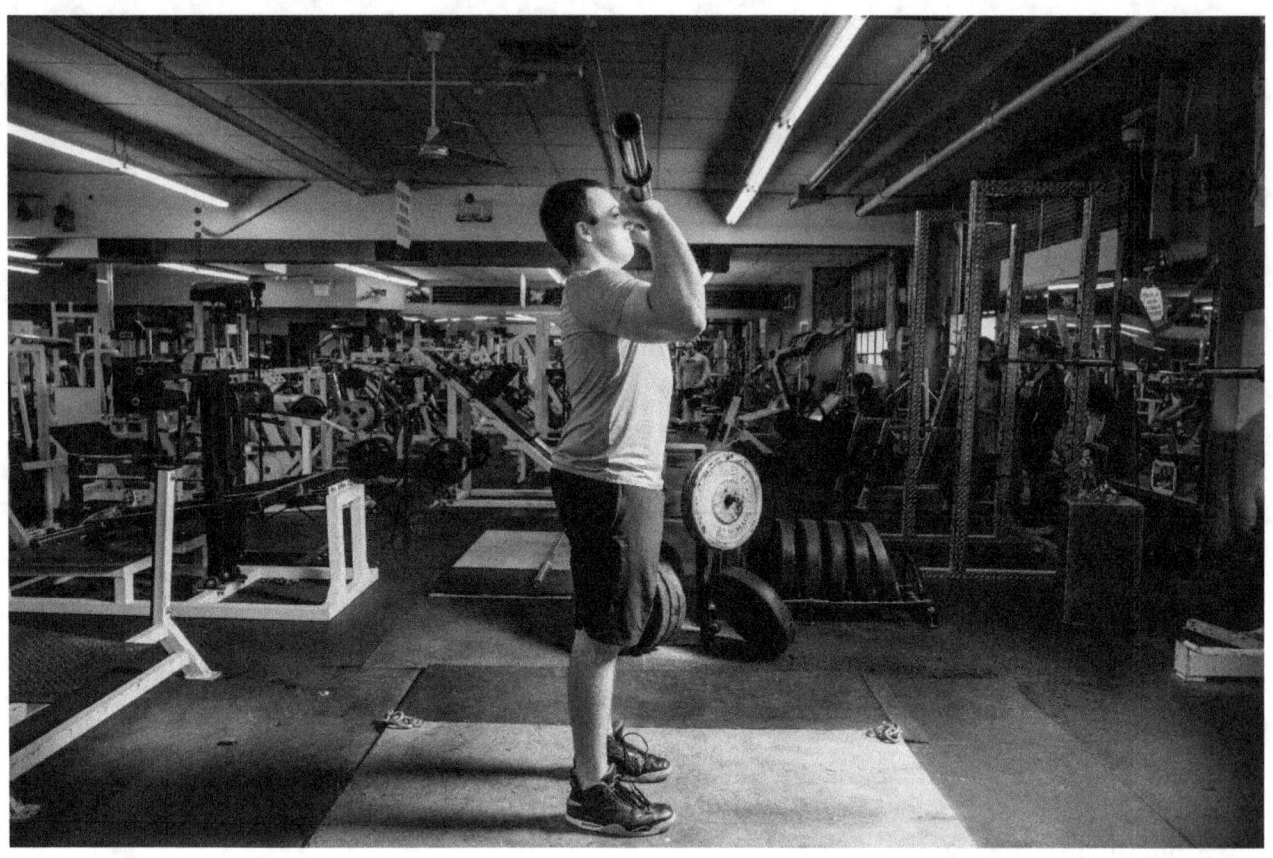

When you have accomplished each of the above, drive the barbell straight up to lockout. Move your head back to clear space for the bar. It's imperative that you keep the bar as close to the midline of your body as possible. When the bar is fully locked out overhead, slowly return the bar to the starting position, as if you were pressing rewind, and repeat for subsequent repetitions.

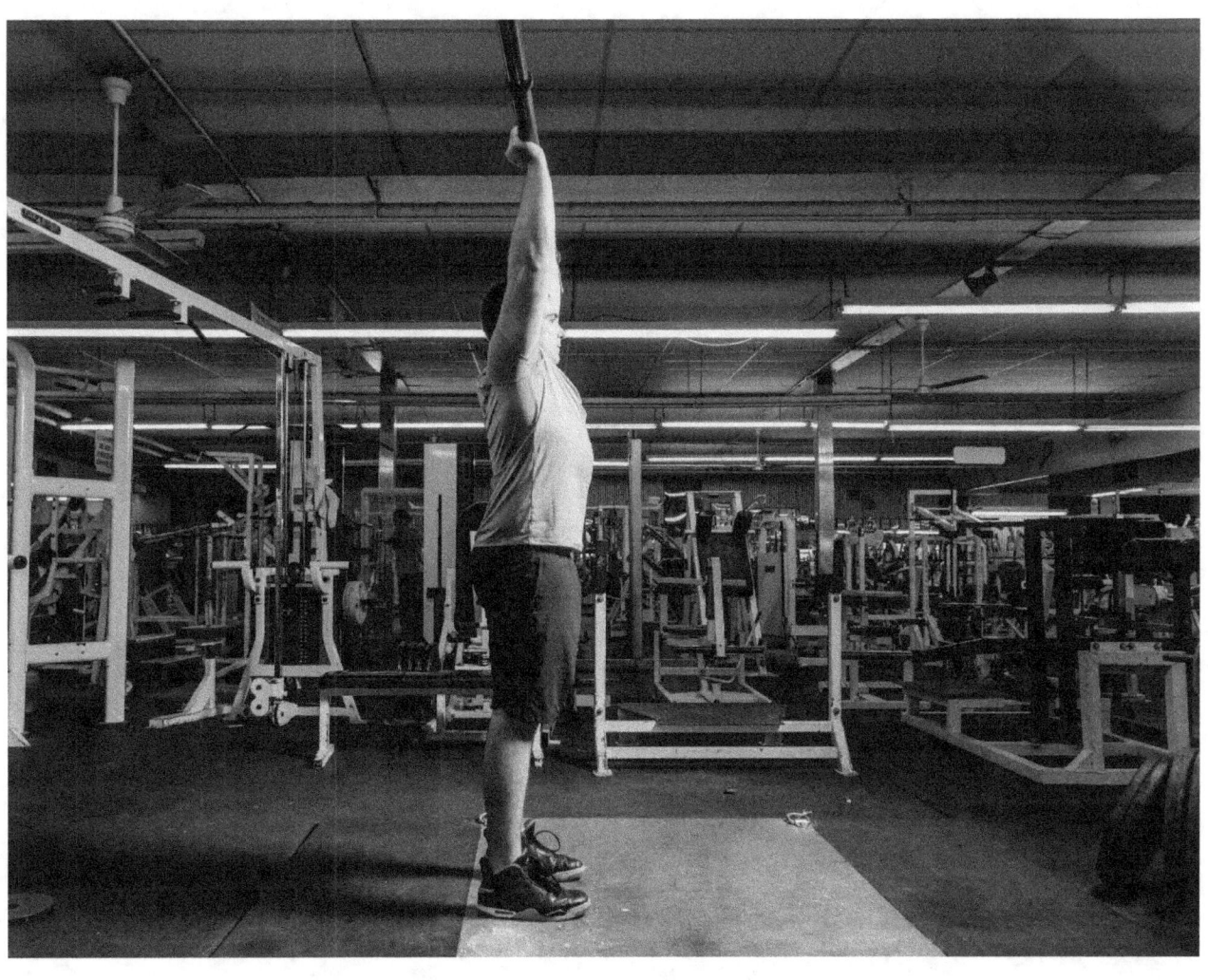

Chapter 5: Organizing The Main Lifts for Long-Term Success

To review, we have admitted that we suck, we have learned that our goal is to execute perfect reps of the squat, bench, deadlift, and press against increasing loads, and we have learned that we are going to use some combination of supplemental and accessory lifts to build the main movement. We also learned that we are going to manipulate volume and intensity to some extent in order to achieve specific adaptations.

Now, at this point, we need to discuss how we program the main lifts, starting from our first day in the gym to potentially elite levels. It is not enough to just come into the gym and try to add more weight every workout. That will eventually lead to stagnation. The solution is periodization, which is a fancy exercise-science term that just means organizing your workouts to reach a specific goal.

Programming the Main Lifts:

The main lift is the most important thing that occurs during the workout. We must be mentally prepared to tackle this lift every training day. Now, the major question is how do we progress on these lifts? The classic example often referenced is Milo of Croton systematically lifting and carrying a bull from its infancy each day, and eventually he was able to lift a full-grown bull. The point of the myth is usually to demonstrate the need for some sort of progressive overload. The point is we don't want to travel in a circle or do random things, we want to be gaining ground every day. By next year, we want to be able to look back and say that we are a lot stronger than we were the year before. However, it is not as simple as just adding weight every workout, if that were the case, then we could lift potentially infinite weights by just increasing the load each time. There is a point where simply adding more weight does not work. However, that does not mean that keeping methods simple and aggressive, especially for a beginner, is a bad thing. It just means that over our careers as trainees we will outgrow certain methods and need to introduce greater complexity in order to keep making progress.

We must organize our training such that the body is subject to greater stress over time, but not such that we overreach and become overtrained. The scientific literature describes this as the General Adaptation Syndrome. The General Adaptation Syndrome describes how the body reacts to stress placed upon it. There are three phases, an alarm phase, a resistance phase, and an exhaustion phase. The alarm phase occurs when the body experiences a novel stress (i.e. a stress greater than that previously applied). This alarm phase may be triggered by using a heavier load than last time, more volume, faster rest periods, etc. What is crucial, however, is that the body **must** be placed under a new stimulus. If you begin by squatting 135 for 5 reps and do that same workout every day for your training career, you will not, after a certain amount of time, trigger an alarm phase because the body is used to that load at that amount of volume. No progression can be made. During the alarm phase, your performance will actually decrease and you will feel sore, etc. This is good because it paves the way for the resistance phase. You break your body down to allow it to build itself back up.

The resistance phase is where the body adapts to the stress you placed upon it and returns to normal functioning. Importantly, however, the body will not just return to its former baseline, it will establish a new, higher baseline marked by neurological adaptation and/or new muscle tissue, allowing for greater performance. This is commonly referred to as "supercompensation." No matter how far you go in training, you must find a way to provide a novel stimulus to the body. This is easy at first but becomes harder the more advanced you get.

The third phase of the General Adaptation Syndrome is the phase we want to avoid, namely the exhaustion phase, which is essentially overtraining. The athlete is unable to recover and performance declines. Note that stressors can be those beyond just the ones induced by weight training. Lack of sleep and poor diet can also create additional stressors. This is why the journey for strength is a 24-hour commitment. If you want to be strong, you have to plan your life accordingly.

Now, I need to digress to make an important point here. A common thing that people say is that you need to have "muscle confusion." And what they interpret that to mean is that you have to do something completely different every few weeks so the body doesn't "adapt." This is a case of a little bit of knowledge being a dangerous thing. You don't have to completely change your workout every week or few weeks to make progress. That's like starting a different major in college every week. You wouldn't get very far in any of them. Instead, you progress within the major, you start with intro classes and eventually to intermediate and then to upper levels. The same is true with training, I can squat every week and make progress by providing a new stimulus to the body in the form of more weight, more reps or less rest, etc.

What I will now provide is a method of programming the main lifts which will result in sensible progression for you. If you are new to training, or have not been seriously committed to the multi-joint, core exercises described above, you should start at the foundations level. And when I say not seriously committed, I mean that you haven't squatted 405 to proper depth, you haven't benched 315 with a pause, and you haven't deadlifted 500. If you haven't done this, start at the Foundations level. Trust me on this, it will help you in the long run. From the Foundations level we will advance to beginner's training, so on and so forth until we reach the elite levels.

Level 1: Foundations

Level 1 I have called the Foundations level because this is where we lay the foundation for strength to develop. If you are anything like me, you are a lifter or athlete who has been taught quite a bit in your life about training, and hardly any of it is right. At the outset, what I want you to do is just get yourself acquainted with the main movements, first with no added resistance or with an unloaded barbell. Refer back to chapter 4 for execution of the main lifts. If you are new to the gym or new to strength training, we are going to start very basic. Here is what I want you to do your first week in the gym:

Day 1 (Monday; Squat):

A) Air Squat or Goblet Squat 5x5 (sets/reps) (you can also begin with air squats and transition into goblet squats)
   - Simply get acquainted with proper bracing: seeking to pull the floor apart with your feet, locking the ribcage down, breathing, and getting the knees out (i.e. generating external rotation in the hips)
   - I start with an air or goblet squat because holding the weight in front of the body allows a less mobile lifter to still achieve proper depth and begin to "feel" the proper execution of the squat
   - As discussed later on, we will then accompany this with some basic accessory work so the lifter can begin to "feel" the legs and build muscle in the areas needed for the squat

Day 2 (Wednesday; Bench Press):

A) Bench Press (empty bar or broomstick) 5x5
   - Again, the focus here is to really begin to feel the proper bracing patterns without having to worry about added resistance just yet. Untrained individuals will likely get a pump just by moving the barbell properly for adequate reps.
   - Again, later when we put everything together we will add assistance exercises to address the prime movers in the bench press

Day 3 (Friday; Deadlift):

A) Deadlift (empty bar—elevated or with light bumper plates if you have access) 5x5
   - The back should be flat and technique should be crisp before you add any additional resistance.

Day 4 (Saturday: Press)

A) Strict Press (empty bar or broomstick) 5x5-8
   - Same rationale here, brace the lower half like the squat, focus on breathing, and on creating tightness by bending the bar and keeping the elbows braced and facing forward. The movement should be perfect before adding resistance.

Now, I know what you are thinking: "Obergfell son, why do you have me working with an empty bar or a broomstick? People at the gym will think it odd." The reason I want you to do this for at least the first week is because I want you to get acquainted with performing the main movements in an effective manner before adding additional variables. We are looking for absolute precision on every rep. Whether you are deadlifting a broomstick or 1000 pounds, we want it to look the same. As you can probably already tell, I am very big on fundamentals. I stress the fundamentals so much because they are the foundation that everything else will be built upon. If you swallow your pride and take the time to do this, you will not be disappointed.

The reason that I do one major lift a day to start is so you can really focus on that one lift for that day. It gives you one big goal to focus on. Then, I will provide you with some isolation work for the muscles involved in the major movement, which we will discuss next. When you are doing the isolation exercises, don't just do them for the sake of doing them, do them to really feel the muscle work. Use a weight that is challenging but one in which you can complete the reps with perfect form. The use of the isolation exercises will give you a better connection with the muscles involved in main movements and will also help build muscle mass, which will then help to add more strength.

Level 2: Beginner

Once you have completed the Foundations phase, we will begin to add weight to the bar. In this phase, for the core lifts (squat, bench, deadlift, strict press), start with a simple 5x5, one that is heavy enough to challenge you but can be completed with perfect form. Each week, you should add 5 pounds, try to beat your 5x5 sets from last week. Remember though, 5 pounds, don't jump the gun. You will repeat this for as long as possible until you can no longer complete a 5x5 set.

When you can no longer complete 5x5 sets on the core lifts, you have a couple options. One option I like is to start by adding weight to the first set only and then dropping down to the weight you previously stalled at for the remaining four sets. Then add a set with the new weight until you get to a 5x5. For example, suppose your last successful 5x5 on the squat was at 225 for 5x5, but then you were unable to complete the 5x5 with 230. What you can do is:

Week 1: 1x5 @ 230, 4x5 @ 225

Week 2: 2x5 @ 230, 3x5 @ 225

Week 3: 3x5 @ 230, 2x5 @ 225

Week 4: 4x5 @ 230, 1x5 @ 225

Week 5: 5x5 @ 230

By breaking it down set by set you allow yourself to continue to make progress week by week, but slow it down so you give yourself time to get more and more comfortable with the previously-challenging weight. As will be clear by the end of the book, I envision strength training as a structure that is both tall and wide. If you shoot up too quickly in just trying to add weight, the structure will collapse because the foundation is not deep enough to support the height. Layering weights in this way ensures that as you build up in weight, your structure is sturdy.

When this layering approach no longer works, you can proceed by adding weight using 3x5 rather than 5x5. This will operate the same way as the 5x5 cycle. Say your last successful 5x5 squat, after the layering approach, was at 275. You can then switch to 280 for 3x5 the following week. Proceed by adding 5 pounds to your 3x5 until you cannot do so any longer. At that point, you can resort to the same layering approach described above, where you add weight to the first set only, then the next week to the first and second set, and then the third week to all three sets. Continue in this way for as long as you can. When you can no longer complete a 3x5, drop it to 3x3.

When that fails, drop down to 3x1 until you reach a true one rep max (1RM) with perfect form. This is the best way to test a true 1RM. Instead of just testing a 1RM on the first day when you are likely wholly unqualified to do so, this approach allows you to gain a degree of proficiency in the lifts before you test, giving you a more accurate, and safer, result. The 1RM you achieve at the end of this cycle can then be used to plug into more advanced programming.

Notice, in accord with the principles we discussed above, this "beginner" block tapers higher volume (5x5) to lower volume, and lower intensity to higher intensity to reach an accurate assessment of your true 1RM. If taken seriously and performed correctly, the Foundations and Beginner cycle can consume a year of training or more. Also, just to make a little more sense of this cycle, you can see from 50,000 feet that at the end of this cycle the lifter, without even knowing it, will have had his or her first rudimentary experience with block periodization. Do you see why?

Now, I want to tie this up to our 50,000 feet chapter so that we can keep a bird's eye view of what's going on here. This beginner's cycle is a rudimentary progression. We stick with sets of 5 because that is a good intermediate number, asking an athlete to perform heavy singles out of the gate is not beneficial to the athlete or the coach. Also, sets of 10 or more tend to become counterproductive because focus can easily be lost when performing higher reps. I want you to really focus on every rep and nail the form down. This progression allows you to do that. With more advanced periodization, every workout depends on you having completed the last one, every workout is a puzzle piece. Here, while that's true to an extent with this system, this system allows you a little more leeway to figure things out as you go. You may discover something about your squat at some point and want to repeat last week's weight because it didn't quite feel right and now you discovered the issue and want to go back. This program allows you to do that. You don't have to add more weight until you are ready. Remember, purge the ego, this is about long term growth and laying the foundation for that growth.

As we discussed above, volume and intensity are inversely correlated. We start with a set number of reps, 5, but we look to increase the weight each week, so therefore our volume, as defined above as (weight x reps x sets=volume load) will increase each week even keeping the reps variable constant. Let me provide an example. Let's say on my first day I achieve a 135 pound squat for 5 sets of 5, volume load=135x5x5, totaling 3375. A week later I come in and achieve a 140 pound squat for 5 sets of 5, volume load now equals 145x5x5, totaling 3500. You see, just by isolating the one variable, to wit the weight, and keeping the rest constant, we still move more volume each week and get stronger.

The next thing I asked you to do was when you can no longer complete sets of 5, to move to sets of three and then sets of 1. Now we are increasing the intensity and actually decreasing volume, remember they are inversely correlated. By lowering the reps, it will allow you to drop some of the volume for the sake of working at higher intensities. For example, imagine that 145 for 5x5 was the best I could do, and the next week I went to 150 for 3x5, volume load now equals 150x3x5=2250, less than the 3500 for the 5x5 at 145. I sacrificed volume to move a heavier load, we are beginning to taper down to higher intensity. This begins to secure neural adaptation and reduces overall fatigue to hit heavier reps. If you can understand this, you are on your way to understanding program design.

Level 3: Intermediate

What I call the "intermediate" phase is where things begin to get more interesting. At this point in our training career, the intensities have become too high to simply continue to add weight to the bar each week. We must begin to rely on different parameters in building the main lifts, which will allow us sufficient time to recover and continue to make progress. The intermediate phase is essentially a more complex progression, in which we begin to add more variables. Instead of keeping the reps constant, we will fluctuate rep ranges and intensities.

Basic intermediate program 1: three-week waves (or linear progression in three intensity zones)

An easy way to begin an intermediate phase is to simply create a repeating three-week wave. To begin the wave, use the 1RM you achieved in your beginner cycle to get started:

Week 1	Week 2	Week 3
3-5x5 @ 70-75%	3-5x3 @ 75-80%	3-5x1 @ 85%

As you can see, this is a very simple method, but more complex than a pure linear progression that we discussed above, to allow you to make continued gains. When you complete a three-week wave, simply increase your max by 5-10 pounds depending on how you feel, and run it over again. Thus, this is more complex than the beginner's cycle because instead of adding 5-10 pounds after every *workout*, we add 5-10 pounds after every *cycle*. This stretches out the progression and allows us to work in multiple intensity zones while still progressing. As you progress through the cycle, what was originally 70-75% is no longer 70-75%, so on and so forth. You are getting stronger by using progressively heavier weights in each three-week wave. A program like this is a perfect segue into more complex periodization. You can think of this as either a percentage-based program or a linear progression across three intensity zones. Again, do you see why?

Now, as we saw in the Beginner's cycle above, we can add complexity to this basic scheme in various ways. First, you can start with three sets and each week add an additional set until you get to five total sets, and then increase your max. Say, for example, you started by running a full three-week cycle with three sets, with a working max of 300. Before having to add weight to your working max, you can, instead, increase the number of sets, making it a nine-week cycle rather than three weeks:

Week 1	3x5 @ 210 (210=70% of 300)
Week 2	3x3 @ 225 (225=75% of 300)
Week 3	3x1 @ 255 (255=85% of 300)
Week 1	4x5 @ 210 (added one set, working max is still 300)
Week 2	4x3 @ 225
Week 3	4x1 @ 255
Week 1	5x5 @ 210
Week 2	5x3 @ 225
Week 3	5x1 @ 255
Week 1 (now up working max to 305 or 310 and start again)	

Another option would be the layering approach we saw above. Let's say that after the last three-week wave you ran with the above cycle, you do not feel that you are ready to progress to another weight for the full number of sets. You can simply increase the weight for the first set and then descend in weight for the subsequent sets. Like so:

Set 1: 215x5

Sets 2-5: 210x5

Next time around you have two choices, you can either add additional sets with 215, or you can continue to increase the first set and have the rest of the sets as slight back down sets. Or, you could combine them and do something like:

Set 1: 215x5

Set 2: 210X5

Set 3-5: 205x5

This is all just about chipping away at heavier weight while also keeping your base wide. As you can see, by layering the weights in this way you will get a lot of work in with 210 (your previous plateau), and as a result will get more and more comfortable with that weight. When you gain confidence and "own" the weight, you then cycle up.

Another great variation on this template is to do what I call repetition ladders. This is a great template to use if you are in a hypertrophy block and want to add muscle. Let's say your program calls for 315 for 5x5 on the squat in week 1. Assume you complete that workout. The next cycle, you will then, on the first set, do 315x6, and then 4x5 at 315. The next cycle after that, 315x7, then 4x5 at 315. You can use this approach to get to whatever number of reps you desire. I would not go beyond 10. You can also stagger the goal to account for the three week wave. Week 1 you may want to shoot for 10 reps, Week 2 shoot for 8 reps, and Week 3 shoot for 6 reps. When you reach your goal, cycle the weight up.

You can go a long way on just a very simple program like this, especially with the choice of proper assistance work. However, the time will ultimately come where you will need to move on to more complex periodization. From this point, the next logical step is clear, namely we just use each week of the three-week block and expand it into longer blocks. The logic is the same, we are just adding complexity.

Basic Intermediate Program 2: Basic Block Periodization

Phase 1: hypertrophy

- Goal: To build muscle mass; to increase technique and control in the main lift.
- Methods: 6-10 rep range, 55-75% of working max

Week 1	Week 2	Week 3
3x10 @ 60%	3x8 @ 65%	3x6 @ 70%

You can use this just as a three-week wave, increasing your training max after each wave and repeating until the desired adaptation is reached, then you can link this up with a strength block.

Or, if you want to get more creative, you can simply up the number of sets each week from 3 to 5 before increasing your working max. This will result in 9 week blocks rather than three-week blocks, as we described above.

The undulating three-week waves, I find, are useful for keeping the training interesting and preventing stagnation that can arise by using the same rep ranges over and over. But from 50,000 feet, what happened here is simply that we isolated a goal, hypertrophy, and, adhering to our principles, namely higher volume and lower intensity, achieved the goal of hypertrophy in a training block.

Now, let's say I've met my hypertrophy goal, and now I want to begin a strength block, where I focus more on honing the mass I have built to be displayed as actual strength.

Phase 2: Strength

- Goal: To begin to hone the newly acquired muscle mass into absolute strength by beginning to work with higher intensities and using slightly lower volume.
- Methods: 75-85% intensity, 4-6 reps.

Week	Sets/Reps	Intensity
1	3x6	75%

2	3x5	80%
3	3x4	85%

Like the other blocks, we can easily make this a 9 week cycle by simply increasing the sets from 3-5 before we increase our working max.

Phase 3: Realization (Peaking)

A realization block can be used to peak for a one-rep max, where you display the hypertrophy and strength developed into one, all-out effort. I like to use 1-3 reps here, to be performed between 85-95%. We will also incorporate a "deload" or an unloading week before attempting a new max.

Week	Reps/Sets	Intensity
1	3x3	85%
2	3x2	90%
3	3x1	95%
4	3x5	60% (deload)
5	MAX	100%+

Once you achieve a new max, take some time off, about a week or so, and then you can begin again with hypertrophy, using the max you achieved as your new working max. That way, you are always progressing and you always know what numbers to use.

What I have illustrated here is a very simple, concise way to organize your training when a simple three-week wave no longer suffices. You can use the same scheme but break the training into separate cycles in order to achieve the required adaptation. When you make it

51

through each of the three phases and achieve a new 1RM, simply take the new 1RM and begin again using that new number.

One more way we can add some complexity to our training is by adding frequency, meaning how often we train the main lifts in a week. The simplest way to do this is to have a "heavy" day and a "light day" or "reps" day, which are performed on different days (with at least two days rest in between). This allows you to keep more volume even as you are moving toward higher intensities. A sample set-up could look like this:

Week	Sets/Reps (Heavy day)	Intensity	Sets/Reps (Reps day)	Intensity
1	3x6	75%	3x10	60%
2	3x5	80%	3x8	65%
3	3x4	85%	3x6	70%

This can be used in repeating patterns, cycling up the working max each time. When switching over to a peaking block, you can either keep the light day light with high reps or make the light day more of an intermediate day:

Week	Reps/Sets	Intensity	Sets/Reps	Intensity
1	3x3	85%	3x10	60%
2	3x2	90%	3x8	65%
3	3x1	95%	3x6	70%

Or

Week	Reps/Sets	Intensity	Sets/Reps	Intensity
1	3x3	85%	3x6	75%
2	3x2	90%	3x5	80%

3	3x1	95%	3x4	85%

The "reps" or "volume" day can be converted to a "speed" day by inverting the sets and reps (rest will still be at least 48 hours between sessions). "Speed" work is ordinarily performed with submaximal loads between 75-85% of your 1 RM, wherein we try to accelerate the barbell (with perfect form!) as fast as possible. This plays on the force=mass x acceleration formula. If we take a maximum lift we can increase our force production by maxing out the mass variable with minimal acceleration, which will increase absolute strength. "Speed" work counterbalances increased acceleration against a mass that is heavy enough to drive up force production. If the weight is too light, you can lift it as fast as you want but you will not get stronger. Why? Because the acceleration multiplied by the minimal mass does not equate to enough force to increase strength.

An example of a concurrent strength and speed cycle is as follows:

Week	Sets/Reps	Intensity	Sets/Reps	Intensity
1	3x6	75%	10x3 (barbell will be moved as fast as possible without compromising form)	60%
2	3x5	80%	8x3 (barbell will be moved as fast as possible without compromising form)	65%
3	3x4	85%	6x3 (barbell will be moved as fast as possible without compromising form)	70%

It is important to me to tie everything back into the 50,000 feet chapter earlier in the book. We are still remaining faithful to our goal of increasing absolute strength on the squat, bench press, deadlift, and press. However, because increasing the load each week is no longer practicable, we are now simply manipulating volume and intensity variables to ensure continued progress and recovery.

Once you have exhausted all progress based on this system (which will actually be a very small number of people), then you may move on to level 4, which is advanced programming.

Level 4: Advanced

I will now go through some advanced techniques that can help you to continue to make progress when you are moving exceptionally heavy poundages on the main lifts. There are a few ways to do this, but the logic is essentially this: we began this book by stating that the main lifts are what we are trying to improve, and the way we did it was by actually performing those main lifts. However, there is a catch, at a certain point (a point where you have become tremendously strong), we shift the logic down one level, meaning that the supplemental exercises become the main movements. By training different movements, namely ones closely resembling the competition lift but not the actual competition lift, the lifter may assure continued progress. These exercises are good because they will provide a novel stimulus and allow you to connect with new muscle fibers that are not activated when performing the main movement. This is helpful because when you activate theses previously dormant motor units, it makes for a better main lift. Moreover, using these special exercises allows you to target weak points in the lift and thereby improve your competition lift. For example, if you are weak off the floor on your competition deadlift, you may want to pull from a deficit for a cycle, this will help you off the floor. If your quads are weak on a squat, you may want to train high bar for a cycle, or perform front squats. It just takes some thought on your part, and this can be very beneficial.

The main way to do this is a twist on the intermediate level program. In any of the methods that were described in the intermediate level, you can simply take them and switch the main movement to address a particular weakness in your training. For example, you may choose to run a cycle using the close stance high bar squat to improve quad strength before returning to an ordinary low-bar back squat cycle. By bringing up the lagging area, you will in turn drive up your ordinary back squat.

At its core, we are dancing around two main issues, the first is the law of accommodation, namely that your response to the same movement will dull over time. On the other hand, the one thing that every personal trainer learns is the SAID principle, specific adaptation to imposed demands. This means that your body will respond to the demands imposed upon it. Thus, if I want to get better at deadlifting, I have to deadlift. Therefore, when we get to advanced levels, we need to find a happy medium between these things. We use exercises that resemble the main lift, but different enough that a novel stimulus is placed on the body, activating new muscle fibers. The drawback to advanced training is essentially that we sacrifice specificity, namely the performance of the main lift. However, such a sacrifice is sensible as by this point, you will have become very proficient in the main lifts. The special exercises represent a novel stimulus and reduce overall stress and fatigue on the body (through modulating intensity). Training with other exercises also reduces the mental stress.

Thus, to get started using an advanced scheme, simply select a special exercise that will target your weak point in the competition movement. I decided to put together a list of special exercises that assist the main lift, and I will share it with you.

Squat	Bench	Deadlift
<ul><li>Box squats</li><li>Front squats</li></ul>	<ul><li>Pause Bench</li><li>Extended pauses</li></ul>	<ul><li>Deficit deadlifts</li></ul>

• All squats versus bands and chains (nearly limitless variety) • High bar squat • Low bar squat • Zercher squats • Squats to low boxes, high boxes, and everything in between • Safety bar squat • Buffalo bar squat • Squats with any specialty bars you have • Reverse band squat • Hex bar deadlifts • Squat from pins (Andersen squats); can be done with various bars • Good morning variations • Hip thrust	• Floor press • Football bar bench • Slingshot bench • Press from pins of different heights (supine, seated, or incline) • Incline press • Military press variations • Close-grip • Wide-grip • Spoto Press • All variations versus bands and chains or both	• Rack pulls from pins at different heights • Deadlift from blocks • Box squats • Conventional deadlift • Sumo deadlift • Hex bar deadlift • Reverse band deadlifts • Good morning variations (suspended, from pins, versus bands, different bars) • Stiff leg deadlifts (from floor and deficit) • Snatch grip deadlift • Zercher deadlift • Power cleans and snatches • All types of deadlifts with bands and chains • Hip thrust

This is just what I could come up with off the top of my head, but the possibilities are really endless. It just comes down to you exposing your weakness in the main lift and using a special exercise to help fix it and recruit new motor units and build new muscle. As a realization block gets closer, switch back, and you will see improvement. At this advanced stage of training, your proficiency in the main lifts is so good that you don't need to train them every day. As long as you are using a similar exercise, you are good.

Chapter 6: Programming Supplemental Lifts

The supplemental lifts, or special exercises, are exercises that are similar to the main lifts and are used to build the main lift. At their core, supplemental movements are used to target weak points, build work capacity, and increase volume so you can continue to make progress on the main lifts. As we previously saw, supplemental lifts can eventually become the main lifts when you reach an advanced stage. This chapter will cover how to use supplemental exercises at each of the four levels: foundations, beginner, intermediate, and advanced.

Supplemental Lifts for the Foundations lifter

The foundations lifter is concerning himself or herself with learning the main movements, thus, there are no real supplemental lifts to do. The foundations level is marked by main movements with no resistance and accessory movements to build the muscles involved with the movement, as will be discussed later. When you are in the foundations phase, focus your attention on learning to execute the main lifts and getting more mentally aware of the muscles and learning to connect with them.

Supplemental Lifts for the Beginner Lifter

When the lifter enters the beginner stage, supplemental lifts will begin to be used. To start, the best way to incorporate supplemental lifts is to simply perform "down sets" of the main movement. This means lowering the intensity and using increased volume to train the main movement further within a training session. To layer this on to our discussion of the beginner phase of the main lift, we can incorporate "down sets" as follows:

- Beginner phase 1: 5x5
  - Day 1: Squat
    - Main Movement: Squat 5x5

- Supplemental movement: Squat 2x10

The same sequence can be used for the other three lifts. I recommend starting your sets of 10 with a weight that is comfortable but challenging, and increase by five pounds each week.

When your main lift progression shifts down to 3x3, you can correspondingly drop the supplemental volume to 6-8 reps per set, while continuing to increase the load. Finally, when you drop down to your 3x1 and singles, the supplemental lifts can correspondingly drop down to sets of 3-5, while continuing to increase the load.

We start simple with the supplemental lifts because, at every stage of the game, we want to continue as far as possible *with the most simple method*. We continue with the most simple method until we can't squeeze another rep out of it, only then do we add complexity.

Supplemental Lifts for the Intermediate Lifter

As the lifter enters the intermediate stage, the supplemental exercises will increase in complexity. The chart I included above regarding advanced training with special exercises is relevant in choosing proper supplemental lifts. For convenience, here is the chart again:

Squat	Bench	Deadlift
<ul><li>Box squats</li><li>Front squats</li><li>All squats versus bands and chains (nearly limitless variety)</li><li>High bar squat</li><li>Low bar squat</li><li>Zercher squats</li><li>Squats to low boxes, high boxes, and everything in between</li><li>Safety bar squat</li><li>Buffalo bar squat</li></ul>	<ul><li>Pause Bench</li><li>Floor press</li><li>Football bar bench</li><li>Press from pins (supine, seated, or incline)</li><li>Slingshot bench</li><li>Incline press</li><li>Military press variations</li><li>Close-grip</li><li>Wide-grip</li><li>Spoto Press</li><li>All variations versus bands and chains or both</li></ul>	<ul><li>Deficit deadlifts</li><li>Rack pulls from pins at different heights</li><li>Deadlift from blocks</li><li>Box squats</li><li>Conventional deadlift</li><li>Sumo deadlift</li><li>Hex bar deadlift</li><li>Reverse band deadlifts</li><li>Good morning variations (suspended, from pins, versus bands, different bars)</li><li>Stiff leg deadlifts (from floor and deficit)</li></ul>

• Squats with any specialty bars you have • Reverse band squat • Hex bar deadlifts • Squat from pins (Andersen squats); can be done with various bars • Good morning variations		• Snatch grip deadlift • Zercher deadlift • Power cleans and snatches • All types of deadlifts with bands and chains

Much like the advanced system above, you should choose a supplemental lift that attacks your weaknesses in the particular lift. I recommend first choosing one supplemental lift that you stick with for an entire cycle, then you may either add another supplemental lift or switch exercises. Proper programming of supplemental lifts is a highly individualized experience, you know best what you need to improve. But don't be overwhelmed, no matter which one or ones you pick, you will be okay because you will begin to recruit new motor units to help build muscle and increase the main lift.

Everyone tends to panic in programming the supplemental lifts, but it does not have to be a stressful experience. The easiest way to program a supplemental movement is simply to have it follow the same general parameters of your main lift. Let's say, for example, that you are running the simple three-week block described at the beginning of the intermediate training discussion, which I will reproduce here:

Week 1	Week 2	Week 3
3-5x5 @ 70-75%	3-5x3 @ 75-80%	3-5x1 @ 85%

In this situation, you have a few options. If you are looking to build more muscle, you can keep the supplemental volume somewhat higher. One thing you can do is choose a rep number such as 8 reps for week one, 6 reps for week two, and 3 reps for week three, and work up to a set on the supplemental lift where you reach the desired number of reps with perfect form but cannot do another rep. Once you complete a three-week cycle, simply increase the weight by five pounds and try to match your goal number. This can continue as long as you continue to make progress on that lift. The advantage of the supplemental lift is that you can swap them out, so you can program them a little more aggressively once progress slows. A sample main lift and supplemental lift using this progression would look like this:

Week 1:

Main Lift (Bench Press): 3-5x5 @ 70%

Supplemental lift (close grip): Work up to heavy set of 8 (keep track of what you get)

Week 2:

Main Lift (Bench Press): 3-5x3 @ 75%

Supplemental lift (close grip): Work up to heavy set of 6 (keep track)

Week 3:

Main Lift (Bench Press): 3-5x1 @85%

Supplemental lift (close grip): work up to a heavy set of 3.

When you conclude this three-week cycle, increase your working max on the main lift and re-run the supplemental cycle trying to beat your numbers from last time by 5-10 pounds. I find this is a fun cycle to run because it provides the opportunity to compete in the gym, even against yourself.

Once progress stalls in that fashion, you can either switch supplemental exercises or you can increase intensity. For example:

Week 1:

Main Lift (Bench Press): 3-5x5 @ 70%

Supplemental lift (close grip): Work up to heavy set of 5 (keep track of what you get)

Accessories

Week 2:

Main Lift (Bench Press): 3-5x3 @ 75%

Supplemental lift (close grip): Work up to heavy set of 3 (keep track)

Week 3:

Main Lift (Bench Press): 3-5x1 @85%

Supplemental lift (close grip): work up to a heavy set of 1 (new record)

When you can no longer establish a new record, swap the exercise and start again with a new one. But keep track of your previous records at each of the rep ranges, and try to beat it next time you use that exercise.

If you would like to be more systematic about things, you can use a percentage-based approach targeted for difference capacities (i.e. hypertrophy, strength, absolute strength). To do this, you will need to test or estimate a working max for the supplemental lift you are planning to use. A simple three-week wave for the deadlift could be:

Week 1:

Main Lift (Deadlift): 3-5x5 @ 70%

Supplemental lift (Deficit Deadlift): 4x6 @ 65%

Week 2:

Main Lift (Deadlift): 3-5x3 @ 75%

Supplemental lift (Deficit Deadlift): 3x6 @ 75%

Week 3:

Main Lift (Deadlift): 3-5x1 @85%

Supplemental lift (Deficit Deadlift): 3x5 @ 85%

You can then add five pounds to your deficit working max and continue the progression. The percentages on the supplemental lift can be adjusted depending on your goal (i.e. lower percentages and higher reps for hypertrophy and higher intensity and lower reps for strength).

Okay, so let's now say that you are moving on to more advanced intermediate programming and you are using a more complex block periodization formula as we discussed above, to wit:

Week 1	Week 2	Week 3
3x10 @ 60%	3x8 @ 65%	3x6 @ 70%

This would be your typical hypertrophy block protocol. In this instance, you have a few options as to supplemental work. The first, as indicated above, would be just to follow the hypertrophy protocol. Pick an exercise and work up to a hard set of 10 in week one, a hard set of 8 in week two, and a hard set of six in week three, and then repeat upping the weight by five pounds and trying to match the desired number of reps.

Another option would be to use the supplemental lift(s) to work different intensities or different capacities. One parameter I really like to use when doing a hypertrophy or high-rep block is use the supplemental lift for "control" work. This includes extended pause benches, "Spoto" press,[2] pause deadlifts, pause squats, box squats, etc. The reason I like that is because it allows you to retain the skill of pausing and controlling a rep without having to work ultra-high intensities. For example, a cycle for bench may be

Exercise	Week 1	Week 2	Week 3
Bench Press	3x10 @ 60%	3x8 @ 65%	3x6 @ 70%
3-second pause bench	4x6 @ 65% (of your 3-second pause max)	3x6 @ 70%	3x6 @ 75%

---

[2] This refers to pausing the bar about an inch off of your chest, and then reversing the weight. They are named after world-record bench presser Eric Spoto.

By using the 3-second pause variation, we can practice the skill of pausing a rep at the bottom while working with higher reps on the main movement. By using the 3-second pause max (a true three seconds, one-Mississippi, two-Mississippi, three-Mississippi, press), it automatically scales the relative intensity down and allows us to be challenged with lighter weights.

Now, when we move on to a strength block for the main lift, to wit:

Week	Sets/Reps	Intensity
1	3x6	75%
2	3x5	80%
3	3x4	85%

In this case, your 3-second pause wave would be:

Week	Sets/Reps	Intensity
1	3x5	80% (of your 3-second pause max)
2	3x4	85%
3	3x3	90%

During the peaking cycle, the supplemental lifts are generally phased out to place the focus on hitting the high intensities on the main lift and reducing overall fatigue for the maximal attempt to come.

You could also use the supplemental lifts to train different intensities on the same day, meaning that you can get some heavier work in by including some heavy movements after the main lift. It is at this point in the cycle I like to use partial lifts. This can be as easy as adding some block pulls after your deadlifts from the floor, board presses to your bench, and partial top half squats or pin squats to your squat day. This is a great way to prime the nervous system to prepare for the heavier work to come. Using a partial range of motion movement also limits nervous system fatigue to keep you fresh for the subsequent weeks. I would recommend jumping up 10% for these movements. A sample block pull cycle could look like this:

Exercise	Week 1	Week 2	Week 3
Deadlift	3x10 @ 60%	3x8 @ 65%	3x6 @ 70%
2-inch block pull	3x6 @ 70% (of your deadlift max)	3x6 @ 75%	3x6 @ 80%

So unlike the 3-second paused bench, in which the performance of the lift scales the intensity down, in this situation the intensity is scaled up by the exercise selection. This is because, in most cases, an individual's max from blocks will be higher than his or her max from the floor. Therefore, using the partials allows for use of heavier weights, which can help get the nervous system prepared for the weights to be used in the strength block and peaking block. This is a systematic way to use partials to feel heavier weights to prime the nervous system throughout a training cycle to move toward a new 1RM. Of course, this same progression could work for board presses on bench or partial squats off the rack.

As you get more and more advanced, you may want to then add an additional supplemental exercise to your program. To take the example of the sample deadlift cycle I provided above, you may want to add pause deadlifts or deficit pulls as well. To do that, simply drop the percentage of the main lift by 10% and perform pause or deficit deadlifts with that weight. For example, week 1 would look like:

A) Deadlift 3x10 @ 60%
B) Block Pull 2x4-6 @ 70%
C) Pause Deadlift or deficit deadlift 2x6 @ 50%

So in that case the deadlift progression (assuming a hypertrophy cycle) would be 60, 65, 70% and reset plus five pounds. The block pull would be 70, 75, 80% and reset plus five pounds. The deficit cycle would be 50, 55, 60% and reset plus five pounds. The percentages would then adjust as you move into the strength cycle. The partial will always be 10% higher, and the extended range of motion movement will be 10% lower. The percentages on the main lift will always be your baseline. Something like this is rather advanced and would require someone with great technique and work capacity to pull off. This type of program should not be used by an unqualified lifter.

Supplemental lifts for the advanced lifter

Now, when the lifter moves on from the intermediate to the advanced stages of training, the supplemental movement will actually become the main movement. We discussed why this is so above, namely because the lifter will be unable to make continuous progress by simply progressing on the main lift, and special exercises will have to be used to correct weaknesses and provide new neural adaptations. You will return to the main movements as you peak for your realization event.

For the advanced lifter, you will still use a supplemental movement, but they will be somewhat further removed than the supplemental lifts for the intermediate lifter (because those movements have now become main movements). Here is a sample menu of supplemental lifts for an advanced lifter.

Squat	Bench	Deadlift
<ul><li>Good morning variations</li><li>Glute ham raises</li><li>Sled pulls</li><li>Belt squats</li><li>Hip thrusts</li><li>Glute Bridges</li><li>Partial ROM Squats</li></ul>	<ul><li>Board presses</li><li>JM Press</li><li>Barbell triceps extension</li><li>Shoulder presses of all sorts</li><li>Spoto Presses of various heights</li></ul>	<ul><li>Good morning variations</li><li>Pendlay rows</li><li>Glute ham raises</li><li>Pulls from blocks greater than 6 inches in height or rack pulls above 6 inches)</li><li>Partial ROM box squats or pin squats</li><li>Barbell hip thrust</li></ul>

If you are running an intermediate-style cycle with a special exercise, simply incorporate the new supplemental exercises in the chart above using the same methods outlined in the intermediate supplemental exercise guide. At the advanced level, the supplemental movement chosen should target weak points. At this level, the key to advancement is to be adept at targeting weak points and making them stronger.

Chapter 7: Programming Accessory Movements

The final level of the pyramid is the accessory work, which are movements that are designed to build muscle mass. These movements, at long last, are similar to your typical bodybuilding movements. These movements help to build the base that builds the main lift. We said in the beginning that a bigger muscle is a *potentially* stronger muscle, meaning that the lifter must not only build muscle but must also train that muscle to be strong, namely in the form of neural adaptation from heavier lifting. When you understand this, you can understand why all three tiers are crucial; no one tier, namely main lift, supplemental lift, or accessory lift is sufficient on its own. In fact, even if you have no interest in raw strength, and you just want to be a bodybuilder or physique competitor, this is the superior way to train, especially if you are natural. Why? Because making strength the priority trains multi-joint movements, which leads to neural adaptation and the nervous system's greater efficiency in recruiting muscle fibers, which makes your bodybuilding work much, much more efficient. Also, building absolute strength will make your accessories stronger. Thus, regardless of your ultimate goal, the training structure proposed in this book is superior.

Accessory exercises are nearly impossible to quantify because there are so many. There are two general principles I want you to keep in mind, then the exploration of these exercises is up to you. The first is that I want you to train the muscles involved in the main movement that you worked on that particular day. Like so:

Day 1 (Squat)

    A) Squat
    B) Supplemental squat or squat variation
    C) Accessories for the quads, hips/hamstrings, back, and abs

Day 2 (Bench Press)

    A) Bench Press

B) Supplemental bench press or bench variation

C) Accessory exercises for the lats, upper back, chest, triceps and biceps

Day 3 (Deadlift)

A) Deadlift

B) Supplemental deadlift or deadlift variation

C) Accessories for abs, lower back, hamstrings, back/traps

Day 4 (Strict Press)

A) Strict Press

B) Supplemental strict press or press variation

C) Accessory exercises for medial delts, rear delts, traps, chest

The second principle, and this cannot be stressed enough, is don't overdo it. This is not an invitation to do a heavy bench press then pile on your favorite bodybuilder's chest workout for the next hour and 45 minutes. I want you to get in the habit of quality over quantity. I'd rather see you do one accessory exercise very well than 5 in a haphazard manner. As a general rule, on these exercises you should be concerned with feeling the muscle and getting a quality contraction on each rep. If this is done right, you won't want to do 10 movements.

You may do as few as 1 and as many as 3 assistance exercises per session. They should be performed, in my opinion, in sets of no less than 8 reps. You may want to go as high as 20-30 reps, even 50 to 100 reps for a shock on pure isolation movements (stack machines or cables). Sets should be between 2-5 sets of 8-20 reps under normal circumstances. Also, you may want to incorporate some intensity techniques for certain lagging muscle groups that you want to bring up. These are your traditional bodybuilding techniques, some of my personal favorites include:

1) Drop sets
2) Forced reps (if you have a reliable training partner only)
3) Three-second eccentrics
4) 10-second rest periods
5) Supersets/giant sets
6) Rest-pause sets

The goal is to get a lot of blood into the muscle. Train the muscle and build it. Using higher reps will also help with recovery.

Below is a chart in which I will list some of my favorite accessory exercises for each of the main lifts. It is not a comprehensive list, it's just my favorites to give you a starting point, then you are free to explore on your own.

Squat	Bench Press	Deadlift	Strict Press
• Safety bar reverse lunges (you can stand on a 2-4 inch box to increase difficulty) • Lunges of all types • Goblet squats • Belt squats • Glute ham raises • Leg extensions • TRX hamstring curls • Regular lying hamstring curls • Unilateral hamstring curls • Leg press (add bands for double the fun) • Hack squats (add bands for double the fun) • Reverse hypers	• JM Press • Rolling DB tri extension • Dips • Assisted dip machine pushdown with a medicine ball • Tri extension with rope, one or both arms • V-grip or straight bar pushdowns • Lat pulldowns (different grips) • Pull-ups of different grips • Seated rows • Bent rows • T-bar rows • DB presses (seated, incline and supine) • Hammer Strength presses • Barbell curl/DB	• Glute ham raise • High rep good mornings with safety squat bar, try bands as well) • Banded good morning • Pull throughs • Chair deadlifts • Reverse hypers • Regular hyperextension • Shrugs with barbell, dumbells or kettlebells • Power shrugs • Barbell hip thrusts	• Lat raises • DB presses (seated, incline and supine) • Rear delt flye (machine and DBs) • Machine presses • Shrugs of all types • Face pulls

	curl/hammer curls		
• Bulgarian split squat • Barbell hip thrust			

As for programming, I believe you should pick your accessory exercises and stick with them throughout a particular training cycle (i.e. no less than three weeks). I don't believe in changing things so frequently that you can never become better at them. Given the variety, you can swap them out when they become stale (after sticking with them for at least one block of training). Keep tabs on the weight you use for a particular exercise and try to beat that weight when you reintroduce the exercise into your program.

Now, for the remainder of this chapter, I will discuss how accessory exercises should be planned for the foundations, beginner, intermediate and advanced lifter.

Accessory exercises for the foundations lifter

The foundations lifter, as discussed above, will concern himself or herself with learning the main lifts and performing relatively simple isolation exercises to begin to exert a degree of control over the muscle and to connect mentally with the muscles involved in the movement. I mentioned above that the first week for a foundations lifter should look like this:

Day 1 (Monday; Squat):

A. Air Squat 5x10 (sets/reps)
B. Lunges with hands folded behind the head 4x8/leg
C. Leg extension 3x10
D. Leg curl 3x10
E. Lying leg raise 3x12
F. Hyperextensions BW (Bodyweight) 3x10-12

Day 2 (Wednesday; Bench Press):

A) Bench Press (empty bar or broomstick) 3-5x5-8
B) Pushups 3x failure (try to increase your number each time)
C) Assisted pullups 3xfailure
D) Assisted dips 3xfailure

E) Seated row 4x15
F) Triceps extension 3x15
G) EZ Curl 3x15

Day 3 (Friday; Deadlift):

A) Deadlift (empty bar) 5x5-8
B) Glute ham raise negatives (simply resist the glute ham raise on the way down and then push yourself back up), these are sometimes known as "Nordic" curls.
C) Hamstring curls 3x10
D) Hyperextensions BW 3x15
E) Kneeling rope crunch 5x10-12

Day 4 (Saturday: Press):

A) Strict Press (empty bar or broomstick) 3x5-8
B) DB front raises 3x10
C) DB Lateral Raises 3x10
D) Rear delt flyes 3x10
E) Shrugs 3x10
F) DB skullcrushers 3x10
G) DB hammer curls 3x10

As you can see, we begin with relatively straightforward, easy to perform accessory exercises for the foundations phase. As the foundations phase only lasts a few weeks, perhaps as little as 1, seldom more than 2-3, simply stick with these particular assistance exercises.

Accessory work for the beginner lifter

The beginner lifter may choose to retain at first the assistance exercises from the foundations phase. When these exercises become stale, the lifter may seek to switch them, however, the lifts should remain relatively basic. Here is a sample list of accessory movements for a beginner:

Shoulders/upper back

1) DB shoulder press
2) Machine pressed (such as a Hammer Strength)
3) Lat raises
4) Machine/DB rear delt flyes

5) Shrugs
6) Face pulls
7) Landmine presses

Lats

I have a somewhat unique rule when it comes to training the lats for a foundations or early beginner lifter, and that rule is that the lifter is **<u>forbidden</u>** from using any row variations with barbells or dumbells until the lifter gains a degree of proficiency in feeling the lats contract with a series of isolation movements. The trouble is that with rows people tend to go way too heavy too soon and get very little lat stimulation, it usually results in jerking the weight and using mostly arms, lower back, etc. This does little other than create poor movement patterns. This is not to say by any means that rows are not excellent, they are. In fact, as you will see below once you begin to be able to "feel" and properly recruit the lats, barbell and dumbbell row variations should be your bread and butter, along with pullups. For a beginner, I would recommend the following progression:

Step 1 (basics):
- Kayak rows
- Straight arm rope pullovers/straight bar pullovers
- Rope cable rows from various heights/angles
- Assisted pullups
- Pulldowns (overhand/underhand)

Step 2 (complexes)
- Assisted pull-up to kayak row
- Straight arm pulldown to kneeling cable row to kneeling pulldowns
- rope pullover to low row

Step 3 (pulldown/pull-up progression)
- Curl bar attachment, under hand grip lat pulldown. Advance to regular, wide-grip lat pulldown
- Assisted pull-up machine, start with a comfortable 10-12 then decrease a plate each session and try to match the reps. Do this until you can complete bodyweight pullups.

Step 4 (regular lats training)
- Unassisted Pull-ups of all grips

- Barbell and DB rows of all types

With this sensible progression, you assure yourself that you will actually have lats, and you will reap the benefits that strong, developed lats bring to the main lifts and your general status in the community.

Arms

There is no reason to overcomplicate arm training. When training the biceps, make sure you stretch and squeeze. When training triceps heavy (i.e. skullcrushers/JM Press), stabilize in accordance with the steps described for the bench press, above.

- Barbell/db/cable curl variations of all types
- Hammer curls
- Triceps pushdown movements of all types
- Rolling DB tri extension
- JM press
- Dips/skullcrushers

Low back/hamstrings

It is better sooner rather than later in your training to develop strong hamstrings and a strong lower back. There is a progression for the hamstrings/low back much like the lats. Don't rush this, be patient and you will be happy you were. If you develop a strong posterior chain, it will serve you for your entire life.

Step 1
- machine hamstring curls
- hyperextensions (bodyweight)
- light reverse hypers
- swiss ball hamstring curls
- glute ham raise negatives
- bodyweight hip thrusts/frog thrusts
- ankle weight hamstring curls (do 20 a day, then 50, then 75, then 100+, just keep breaking your record, this is excellent restoration work)

Step 2
- TRX hamstring curls
- Weighted hyperextensions

- Heavier and more frequent reverse hypers
- Band good mornings
- Pull-throughs
- Band-assisted glute ham raises
- Band resisted hip thrusts
- Ankle weight hamstring curls

Step 3
- Glute-ham raises (first put your arms behind you, then arms in front of you)
- Heavy reverse hypers
- Heavier hyperextensions/"Deadlift" hyperextensions where you stabilize the posterior chain and lats and perform a barbell deadlift while on the hyperextension bench
- Barbell hip thrusts (this exercise is now infinitely loadable, making it a good supplemental choice for the intermediate/advanced lifter)
- Good morning variations for high and intermediate reps (I like the safety squat bar the most for these)

Step 4
- Glute ham raise from a decline/weighted/versus bands (Jedi status)
- RDLs
- Stiff leg deadlifts
- Heavier good mornings
- Heavy barbell hip thrusts/glute bridges

Much like the lats, you must first be able to feel the hamstrings work, get in touch with them mentally, this will serve you when you go on to do more complex exercises. The beginner phase allows you to start with more simple exercises and build your way up. By doing things this way, you will get a lot out of movements like stiff leg deadlifts and good mornings, exercises that many people butcher because they never learned to effectively recruit the hamstrings.

Abs

Abdominal/core training can take a variety of forms and is also crucial for all lifters/athletes. Everyone must have a strong core, you cannot be strong without it. I break abdominal training into crunching varieties, anti-rotational (resisting rotation), static, rotational training, and direct oblique work. The beginner should start with bodyweight exercises to learn to feel the abdominals working. Remember, when we are working the abdominals we actually want to work the abdominals, not the hip flexors, which tend to take over when athletes get sloppy doing ab work. Thus, let's look at a good ab progression for the beginner as he or she moves up the ranks of training.

Step 1 (train 1-3 exercises per day, be more concerned with quality rather than quantity, start with two sets per exercise and then build up to 4 per exercise, when you can do three exercises for 4 sets of at least 20, you may move on to step 2); very little if any rest period should be taken:
- Basic crunches
- Lying leg raises
- Oblique crunches
- Reverse crunches
- Planks (start with 3 sets for 30 seconds and go from there, remember squeeze the core the entire time on these)
- Side planks (same as for regular planks, except you will start with 30 seconds per side)
- Bicycles (should be performed properly with full stretch and full contraction)
- Russian twists

Step 2
- Decline sit-ups
- Hanging leg raise (first knees then legs straight out)
- Oblique DB side bends
- Ab wheel rollouts (start from the knees)
- Weighted planks (start with a 25 plate)
- Weighted Russian twist
- Med ball throws (slams, rotational throws, tornado ball)
- Pallof press (vertical and horizontal)
- Busdrivers
- floorwipers

Step 3
- Hanging windshield wipers
- Rollouts from a standing position
- Glute ham raise sit ups (can incorporate bands or weight)
- TRX fallouts
- Stir the pot
- Heavy planks
- Sledgehammer work
- Weighted hanging leg raises

Once again, as is the theme of the entire book, start simple and progress when ready. Remember, there is no time limit on this. Progress slowly and surely, and you will reach your destination. Many people want to go straight to the top and end up burning out. Remember our principles, 1% better than the last workout, that can mean an additional set, an additional rep, more weight, more complexity. You can't do a hanging windshield wiper before you can do a simple hanging leg raise, in the same way you can't do algebra without first taking basic math. If you remain steadfast, you will get there.

Quads

I call this section "quads," but in reality most of these lower body movements will incorporate the quad, hamstrings, and hips. There are many options when it comes to accessories for the quads. I generally like to incorporate a squat-type movement (belt squat or hacks), then do a single-leg movement, and finish with something like leg extension or a sled push/drag.

- Belt squat
- Sled pushes/drags
- Leg press
- Hack squats
- Leg extension
- Lunges of all sorts (barbell, DB, safety bar, forward, reverse, lateral)
- Bulgarian split squats (start unweighted)
- Step ups

Chest

The chest is another area where people tend to lag because people end up compensating significantly with other joints/muscle groups. That is why many times people will do a great deal of pressing with very little chest development. If you bench correctly, as described above, you will be well on your way to building a solid chest. However, in terms of foundations/beginner work, I like to start simple and give the chest a chance to succeed.

Step 1
- Bodyweight pushups (or assisted pushups if necessary)
- Assisted dips
- Flye variations (machine, cable)-the key here is to keep the tension on the chest the entire time, the flye movement reduces the chance of recruiting things other than the chest, but you still have to focus.
- Machine presses

Step 2
- Weighted or band-resisted pushups
- DB presses (incline, flat, decline)
- DB flyes
- Dips

Laying the foundation as described above will help you to recruit the chest more on the free weight pressing exercises.

Accessory work for the Intermediate/advanced lifter

As seen in the section above, the lifter in the beginner phase will start will simple movements and begin using more complex accessory work as the lifter gains more proficiency. The progressions outlined above, if done correctly, will likely outlive the beginner phase and extend into the intermediate phase. Thus, even if you have entered the intermediate phase, continue to follow the progressions outlined above until you get to the end. From there, the intermediate and advanced lifter may use these exercises to continue to build muscle. The exercises chosen should be increasingly chosen to target and strengthen lagging muscle groups. The biggest difference between the beginner and the intermediate/advanced lifter is the ability to self-assess. The foundations/beginner lifter is concerned primarily with strengthening everything and building muscle generally, whereas the intermediate/advanced lifter needs to be adept at targeting weaknesses in order for continued progression to take place. Finally, intermediate and advanced lifters may seek to use more intensity techniques described above than the foundations and beginner lifter (to wit drop sets, forced reps, 10-second rest periods, supersets and giant sets). Incorporating the specialty techniques described above allow the lifter to complete more work in less time. As the lifter begins to get into shape, he or she will be able to shorten rest periods and complete more work. Eventually, the high intermediate/advanced lifter may want to begin to incorporate more volume in the form of smaller workouts outside of the main training session as his or her work capacity increases.

Chapter 8: Organizing Training Blocks

To review, I have taken you step-by-step through the theory of the program, why and how it works, how to perform the main lifts, and how to program your main lifts, supplemental movements, and accessory movements from start to finish. You already know everything you need to know to be strong. However, I know many people will want to see all of this practically applied in one place. So here is my plan, let's take a hypothetical lifter who has no training experience, and we will start him/her off at the foundation phase and build him/her up to an elite level. This is a sample program, just to show you how these variables fit together and how we can put them together through each phase of the program.

Step 1: Foundations

Hypothetical decides to get strong and muscular. Hypothetical lifter has horsed around in the gym a little, maybe a few cable curls and crunches here and there. Hypothetical lifter will start at the foundations phase. Here is hypothetical lifter's first week of training:

Day 1 (Monday; Squat):

    A) Air Squat 5x10 (sets/reps)
    B) Lunges with hands folded behind the head 4x8 steps/leg
    C) Leg extension 3x10
    D) Leg curl 3x10
    E) Lying leg raise 3x12
    F) Hyperextensions BW (Bodyweight) 3x10-12

Day 2 (Wednesday; Bench Press):

    A) Bench Press (empty bar or broomstick) 3-5x5-8
    B) Pushups 3x failure
    C) Assisted pullups 3xfailure
    D) Assisted dips 3xfailure
    E) Seated row 4x15
    F) Triceps extension 3x15
    G) EZ Curl 3x15

Day 3 (Friday; Deadlift):

A) Deadlift (elevated empty bar) 5x5-8
B) Glute ham raise negatives/Nordic curl (simply resist the glute ham raise on the way down and then push yourself back up)
C) Hamstring curls 3x10
D) Hyperextensions BW 3x15
E) Kneeling rope crunch 5x10-12

Day 4 (Saturday: Press):

A) Strict Press (empty bar or broomstick) 3x5-8
B) DB front raises 3x10
C) DB Lateral Raises 3x10
D) Rear delt flyes 3x10
E) Shrugs 3x10
F) DB skullcrushers 3x10
G) DB hammer curls 3x10

Hypothetical lifter will use this phase to master the techniques described in chapter 5 and will become comfortable executing the main lifts with no added resistance. Hypothetical lifter will also begin some basic isolation exercises to start building the muscle and creating a neural connection with the muscles, as well as building work capacity. Hypothetical lifter may choose to move on after one week if he/she is feeling pretty good about executing the main lift, or he/she may choose to repeat this week once or even twice. The key is to make sure you have the main movements down.

Step 2: Beginner Phase for Hypothetical Lifter

After the 1-3 weeks (or more if necessary) spent in the foundation phase, Hypothetical lifter will now begin training with a loaded barbell. On the first day of loaded barbell training, Hypothetical lifter performs the core lifts with an unloaded barbell for a set of 5 and proceeds to work up to a set of 5 for that day that he can complete with perfect form, and will complete five total sets. Hypothetical lifter errs on the side of starting too light to ensure that technique is maintained. Hypothetical lifter is not concerned with starting too light initially because hypothetical lifter has committed to being strong for his or her lifetime, not just for six weeks or six months. Hypothetical lifter knows the importance of laying a proper foundation. Hypothetical lifter begins the following beginner training block:

Day 1: Squat

A) Squat 5x5 (with perfect form)
B) Barbell lunges 4x6-8 steps per leg (NOTE: for a relatively new lifter I like the barbell variation because chances are it will require the lifter to stay upright and use the legs. Too often with dumbbell lunges the torso will drift forward as the tiring lifter seeks to rely more on the back)
C) Leg curl 3x10-12

C1) Goblet squat 3x12

Abs (3 rounds):

A) Plank (30 seconds)
B) Side plank (each side 30 seconds)

Conditioning: Prowler/sled pushes, or hill sprints

Day 2: Bench Press

A) Bench Press 5x5 (with perfect form)
B) Pushups (bodyweight or with added resistance) 50 total in as few sets as possible
C) DB flyes 3x15
D) Kayak Rows 3x8/side
E) Rope pullover to kneeling pulldown 3x10, rest only after superset is complete
F) V-bar pushdown 4x20
G) Barbell curl 4x10

Day 3: Deadlift

A) Deadlift 5x5 (with perfect form)
B) Band assisted glute ham raises 3x5-8
C) Weighted hyperextensions 3x10-12
D) Straight arm pullover 4x15

D1) EZ Curl bar underhand grip lat pulldown 4x10-12

Abs (4 rounds):

A) Basic crunch (20 seconds)
B) Lying leg raise (20 seconds)
C) Oblique crunch (20 seconds/side)

Day 4: Strict Press

A) Strict Press 5x5 (with perfect form)
B) One-arm landmine press 3x10-12
B1) Band pull-aparts 3x25
C) Rope face pulls 4x25
C1) Lateral raises 4x12-15
D) EZ bar skullcrushers to close grip press 3x10, rest between supersets
E) DB curl to DB Hammer Curl 3x8 each

The illustration above shows the application of the principles described in the above chapters. Hypothetical lifter begins the 5x5 progression on the main lift, and relies on basic accessory exercises to begin connecting with and building the muscles involved in the main movements. The main focus here is on that first 5x5 set, which is the most important aspect of the workout. As you can see, for the accessory work hypothetical lifter is using the progressions that I have laid out in the accessory lifts chapter. You can see that during the foundations phase, for example, hypothetical lifter was using glute-ham raise negatives as the primary accessory. After a few weeks, when hypothetical lifter began the beginner phase, the exercise increased in complexity to full range of motion glute ham raises with band assistance. Your progression will be dependent on you and how you feel with the particular exercise. If you have to carry over performing just negatives on the glute ham raise into the beginner phase, that is not a problem. Progress at your own speed, it's not a race. It's about quality.

Now, suppose hypothetical lifter has been progressing on his or her 5x5 and wants to add in more volume on the main lifts to keep the progress going for as long as possible. Hypothetical lifter begins to incorporate "down sets":

Day 1: Squat

A) Squat 5x5; 2x8-10 (for the down sets, hypothetical lifter begins light and uses a weight at which both sets are challenging but can be done with perfect form, and progresses from there)
B) DB Bulgarian split squat 4x8/leg
C) TRX hamstring curls 4x8
D) Landmine squats 3x10

D1) DB Step-ups 3x12

Abs:

1) Floorwipers 3x10/side
2) Swiss ball "stir the pot" 3x10/side
Conditioning

Day 2: Bench Press

A) Bench Press 5x5; 2x8-10 (for the down sets, hypothetical lifter begins light and uses a weight at which both sets are challenging but can be done with perfect form, and progresses from there)
B) DB Incline Press 4x8-10
B1) Band pull-aparts 4x30
C) Pull-ups 3xfailure
C1) Face pulls 4x30
D) Chest supported DB row 3x10
E) Barbell curl 4x12
F) DB rolling extension 3x8
F1) band pushdown 3x20

Day 3: Deadlift

A) Deadlift 5x5; 2x8-10 (for the down sets, hypothetical lifter begins light and uses a weight at which both sets are challenging but can be done with perfect form, and progresses from there)
B) Safety bar good mornings 4x12-15
C) Band-resisted hip thrusts 4x20
D) Shrugs 4x20

Abs:

A) Standing pallof press 3x30 sec/side
B) Decline sit ups 3x10

Finisher: 100 swiss ball crunches

Day 4: Strict Press

A) Military Press 5x5; 2x8-10 (for the down sets, hypothetical lifter begins light and uses a weight at which both sets are challenging but can be done with perfect form, and progresses from there)
B) DB Arnold Press 4x8-10
B1) Machine rear delt flye 4x20
C) Lat raise (50 total in as few sets as possible)
D) Rear delt DB swing (50 total in as few sets as possible)
E) EZ cable curl (100 reps in as few sets as possible)
F) V-bar pushdown (100 reps in as few sets as possible)

So here we see that hypothetical lifter has added additional volume in the form of down sets to the main lifts. This is now the beginnings of incorporating "supplemental" work into the program. We can also see that now that the lifter is becoming more advanced, the lifter is using more complex accessory movements. However, since the lifter is still not extensively experienced, the accessory work has not reached the pinnacle of complexity. For example, the lifter is using a chest supported dumbbell row to begin becoming comfortable with free weight rowing movements, but is using the chest support to allow for greater focus on the back. There is no completely free rowing such as standing barbell or T-bar rows yet, as the lifter is still building up to them.

Now suppose that hypothetical lifter has completed a 5x5 with 315 on the squat, a 5x5 with 225 on the bench, a 5x5 with 315 on the deadlift, and a 5x5 with 135 on the military press, and the lifter cannot complete a 5x5 with the next required weight. It is at this point that the lifter can then rely on the layering approach to continue progress at the "5s" level:

Day	Week 1	Week 2	Week 3	Week 4	Week 5
Squat	Main work: 325x5 315 4x5	Main work: 325 2x5 315 3x5	Main work: 325 3x5 315 2x5	Main work: 325 4x5 315 1x5	Main work: 325 5x5 Down sets: 2x8-10

	Down sets: 2x8-10	Down sets: 2x8-10	Down sets: 2x8-10	Down sets: 2x8-10	1-3 accessory exercises for the legs/back/abs
	1-3 accessory exercises for the legs/back/abs	1-3 accessory exercises for the legs/back/abs	1-3 accessory exercises for the legs/back/abs	1-3 accessory exercises for the legs/back/abs	
Bench Press	Main work: 235x5 225 4x5 Down sets: 2x8-10 1-3 accessory exercises for the back/chest/ arms	Main work: 235 2x5 225 3x5 Down sets: 2x8-10 1-3 accessory exercises for the back/chest/ arms	Main work: 235 3x5 225 2x5 Down sets: 2x8-10 1-3 accessory exercises for the back/chest/ arms	Main work: 235 4x5 225 1x5 Down sets: 2x8-10 1-3 accessory exercises for the back/chest/ arms	Main work: 235 5x5 Down sets: 2x8-10 1-3 accessory exercises for the back/chest/ arms
Deadlift	Main work: 325x5 315 4x5 Down sets: 2x8-10 1-3 accessory exercises for the legs/back/abs	Main work: 325 2x5 315 3x5 Down sets: 2x8-10 1-3 accessory exercises for the legs/back/abs	Main work: 325 3x5 315 2x5 Down sets: 2x8-10 1-3 accessory exercises for the legs/back/abs	Main work: 325 4x5 315 1x5 Down sets: 2x8-10 1-3 accessory exercises for the legs/back/abs	Main work: 325 5x5 Down sets: 2x8-10 1-3 accessory exercises for the legs/back/abs
Military Press	Main work: 145x5 135 4x5 Down sets: 2x8-10 1-3 accessory movements	Main work: 145 2x5 135 3x5 Down sets: 2x8-10 1-3 accessory movements	Main work: 145 3x5 135 2x5 Down sets: 2x8-10 1-3 accessory movements	Main work: 145 4x5 135 1x5 Down sets: 2x8-10 1-3 accessory movements	Main work: 145 5x5 Down sets: 2x8-10 1-3 accessory movements for the

	for the shoulders/up per back/arms	for the shoulders/up per back/arms	for the shoulders/up per back/arms	for the shoulders/up per back/arms	shoulders/up per back/arms

When hypothetical lifter completes this block, he/she moves up to the next weight. One more important point, for purposes of convenience I assumed that all four lifts stalled at the same time. This will not always happen in real life. Many times one lift will stall before the others. In most situations, I find that the upper body lifts will stall more quickly than the lower body lifts. If that's the case, it is fine to stagger the programming. Move on to more advanced programming for the lifts that are stalling and keep maximizing your barbell for the lifts that are not. The shortest distance between two points is a straight line, don't deviate from that until you have to.

Now assume that the lifter has stalled with his 5s progression, even with the layering approach, and now seeks to cycle down to the 3x3 wave:

Day 1: Squat

A) Squat 3x3; 2x6-8 (remember, the lifter will also cycle down the down sets as he or she approaches a true 1 RM, but will add weight)
B) Pause squat 3x5
C) Leg press (Up to a heavy set of 20 and then drop set)
D) Ham curls 4x40, 30, 20, 10 increasing weight each time

Abs:

1) Half-kneeling cable chop 3x10/side
2) Standing pulldown abs 3x25

Conditioning

Day 2: Bench Press

A) Bench Press 3x3; 2x6-8 (remember, the lifter will also cycle down the down sets as he or she approaches a true 1 RM, but will add weight)
B) Close-grip bench 3x5
B1) Band pull-aparts 4x30
C) Pull-ups 3xfailure
C1) Face pulls 4x30

D) T-bar rows 4x10-12

E) Barbell curl 4x12

F) Skullcrushers to pullovers to press 3x10

Day 3: Deadlift

A) Deadlift 3x3; 2x6-8 (remember, the lifter will also cycle down the down sets as he or she approaches a true 1 RM, but will add weight)

B) Pause deadlift 3x5

C) Safety bar good mornings 4x12-15

E) Barbell hip thrusts 4x20

F) Shrugs 4x20

Abs:

C) Standing pallof press 3x30 sec/side

D) Weighted decline sit ups 3x10

Day 4: Strict Press

A) Military Press 3x3; 2x6-8 (remember, the lifter will also cycle down the down sets as he or she approaches a true 1 RM, but will add weight)

B) Incline press 3x5

B1) Cable rear delt flye 4x20

C) Lat raise 4x40, 30, 20, 10 then 10, 20, 30, 40 increasing each time then decreasing each time on the way back up

D) Face pulls (100 reps in as few sets as possible)

E) Biceps/triceps

Now you can see that the lifter has cycled down to 3x3 and has also cycled the down sets down to 6-8 reps per set. Notice also that the lifter has added a supplemental movement as well on each day to assist in continuing to build the main movement. The lifter has also added complexity to the accessory movements in the form of more complex exercises (i.e. the T-bar row), and also more intensity techniques such as ladder sets, drop sets, and 100 rep sets. This provides an example of how a lifter will progress on the main, supplemental, and accessory lifts.

The lifter can then use the layering approach on the 3x3 as described above to make as much progress as possible. When the noticeably thicker hypothetical lifter finishes this cycle, he/she can then take a true 1RM in the squat, deadlift, bench press, and strict press. These will represent an accurate assessment of hypothetical lifter's true 1RM. From that point, he/she will begin his intermediate programming, using a working max of 90-95% of the 1RM achieved at the end of the beginner phase.

Intermediate Phase for Hypothetical Lifter

When hypothetical lifter can no longer make progress using this standard week-by-week progression, he/she will start to organize the training into longer blocks, rather than just workout to workout. The lifter will also begin to manipulate volume and intensity variables to ensure sufficient recovery and progress. Let's say that hypothetical lifter identified quad strength as an issue on the squat, chest as an issue on the bench, and hamstrings as an issue on the deadlift. Hypothetical lifter begins the following intermediate cycle:

	Week 1	Week 2	Week 3
Squat	Main work: 5x5 @ 70% Supplemental work Front Squat 4x8-10 (start with a comfortable weight that is taxing but allows the reps to be properly performed) Accessory work for the quads first and then hamstrings, back, glutes and/or abs	Main work: 5x3 @ 77.5% Supplemental work Front Squat 4x6-8 (slightly greater load than last week but same goal, taxing weight but generally comfortable) Accessory work for the quads first then hamstrings, back, glutes and/or abs	Main work: 5x1 @ 85% Supplemental work Front Squat 4x3-6 (same deal) Accessory work for the quads first then hamstrings, back, glutes and/or abs
Bench Press	Main work: 5x5 @ 70% Supplemental work: Wide-grip bench 4x8-10 (start with a comfortable weight that is taxing but	Main work: 5x3 @ 77.5% Supplemental work: Wide-grip bench press 4x6-8 (slightly greater load, same principles)	Main work: 5x1 @ 85% Supplemental work: Wide-grip bench press 4x3-6

	allows the reps to be properly performed) Accessory work for the chest first then the other applicable muscle groups	Accessory work for the chest first then the other applicable muscle groups	Accessory work for the chest first then the other applicable muscle groups
Deadlift	Main work: 5x5 @ 70% Supplemental work: Stiff-leg deadlift 4x8-10 Accessory movements for the hamstrings first then other applicable muscle groups	Main work: 5x3 @ 77.5% Supplemental work: Stiff-leg deadlift 4x6-8 Accessory movements for the hamstrings first then other applicable muscle groups	Main work: 5x1 @ 85% Supplemental work: Stiff-leg deadlift 4x3-6 Accessory movements for the hamstrings first then other applicable muscle groups
Military Press	Main work: 5x5 @ 70% Accessory work for the shoulders, traps, and arms	Main work: 5x3 @ 77.5% Accessory work for the shoulders, traps, and arms	Main work: 5x1 @ 85% Accessory work for the shoulders, traps, and arms

When hypothetical lifter finishes a cycle, he increases his working max by 5-10 pounds and then resets. From there, the lifter used a supplemental lift to attack the particular weaknesses outlined above which were discovered during the beginner's cycle, and used accessory movements to target the weak muscle group before moving on to stronger muscle groups. Once the three-week cycle has been completed, the lifter can choose to continue with the same supplemental exercises if he/she continues to improve. The lifter may also stick with the same accessory paradigm if there is more work to be done in bringing up that lagging muscle group.

Or, if the lifter feels the weakness has been addressed he or she may choose to attack a different body part with either a new supplemental lift or new accessories.

Let us now assume that after a year or two of basic intermediate training as outlined above, hypothetical lifter needs to increase complexity to keep making progress. At this point, hypothetical lifter has far surpassed almost everyone in his gym, and the patrons are asking him what his supplement stack is. Hypothetical lifter is amused by this because he has just been training using the basic, sound principles already discussed and has been eating to fuel his performance. Hypothetical lifter then draws up the following intermediate cycle, using his current training max to base all percentages off of:

PHASE 1: Hypertrophy (6 weeks, i.e. two cycles)

	Week 1	**Week 2**	**Week 3**
Squat	Main work: 3x10 @ 60%	Main work: 3x8 @ 65%	Main work: 3x6 @ 70%
	Supplemental lift #1: Reverse band squat 3x10 @ 70%	Supplemental lift #1: Reverse band squat 3x8 @75%	Supplemental lift #1: Reverse band squat 3x6 @ 80%
	Supplemental lift #2 Pause Squat 2x8 @ 50%	Supplemental lift #2: Pause Squat 2x6 @ 55%	Supplemental lift #2: Pause Squat 2x4 @60%
	Accessory work to target weakness/for symmetry	Accessory work to target weakness/for symmetry	Accessory work to target weakness/for symmetry
Bench Press	Main work: 3x10 @ 60%	Main work: 3x8 @ 65%	Main work: 3x6 @ 70%
	Supplemental lift #1: Slingshot bench 3x10 @ 70%	Supplemental lift #1: Slingshot bench 3x8 @75%	Supplemental lift #1: Slingshot bench 3x6 @ 80%
	Supplemental lift #2: 3-second pause bench 2x8 @ 50%	Supplemental lift #2: 3-second pause bench 2x6 @ 55%	Supplemental lift #2: 3-second pause bench 2x4 @60%

	Accessory work to target weakness/for symmetry	Accessory work to target weakness/for symmetry	Accessory work to target weakness/for symmetry
Deadlift	Main work: 3x10 @ 60% Supplemental lift #1: 4-inch block pull 3x10 @ 70% Supplemental lift #2: Deficit deadlift 2x8 @ 50% Accessory work to target weakness/for symmetry	Main work: 3x8 @ 65% Supplemental lift #1: 4-inch block pull 3x8 @75% Supplemental lift #2: Deficit deadlift 2x6 @ 55% Accessory work to target weakness/for symmetry	Main work: 3x6 @ 70% Supplemental lift #1: 4-inch block pull 3x6 @ 80% Supplemental lift #2: Deficit deadlift 2x4 @60% Accessory work to target weakness/for symmetry
Military Press	Main work: 3x10 @ 60% Accessory work for the shoulders, traps, and arms	Main work: 3x8 @ 65% Accessory work for the shoulders, traps, and arms	Main work: 3x6 @ 70% Accessory work for the shoulders, traps, and arms

PHASE 2: Strength (6 weeks, i.e. two cycles)

Squat	Main work: 3x6 @ 75% Supplemental lift #1: Reverse band squat 3x6 @ 80% Supplemental lift #2 Pause Squat 2x6 @ 65% Accessory work to target weakness/for symmetry	Main work: 3x5 @ 80% Supplemental lift #1: Reverse band squat 3x5 @ 85% Supplemental lift #2: Pause Squat 2x5 @ 70% Accessory work to target weakness/for symmetry	Main work: 3x4 @ 85% Supplemental lift #1: Reverse band squat 3x3 @ 90% Supplemental lift #2: Pause Squat 2x3 @75% Accessory work to target weakness/for symmetry
Bench Press	Main work: 3x6 @ 75%	Main work: 3x5 @ 80%	Main work: 3x4 @ 85%

	Supplemental lift #1: Slingshot bench 3x6 @ 80%	Supplemental lift #1: Slingshot bench 3x5 @85%	Supplemental lift #1: Slingshot bench 3x3 @ 90%
	Supplemental lift #2: 3-second pause bench 2x6 @ 65%	Supplemental lift #2: 3-second pause bench 2x5 @ 70%	Supplemental lift #2: 3-second pause bench 2x3 @75%
	Accessory work to target weakness/for symmetry	Accessory work to target weakness/for symmetry	Accessory work to target weakness/for symmetry
Deadlift	Main work: 3x6 @ 75%	Main work: 3x5 @ 80%	Main work: 3x4 @ 85%
	Supplemental lift #1: 4-inch block pull 3x6 @ 80%	Supplemental lift #1: 4-inch block pull 3x5 @85%	Supplemental lift #1: 4-inch block pull 3x3 @ 90%
	Supplemental lift #2: Deficit deadlift 2x6 @ 65%	Supplemental lift #2: Deficit deadlift 2x5 @ 70%	Supplemental lift #2: Deficit deadlift 2x3 @75%
	Accessory work to target weakness/for symmetry	Accessory work to target weakness/for symmetry	Accessory work to target weakness/for symmetry
Military Press	Main work: 3x6 @ 75%	Main work: 3x5 @ 80%	Main work: 3x4 @ 85%
	Accessory work for the shoulders, traps, and arms	Accessory work for the shoulders, traps, and arms	Accessory work for the shoulders, traps, and arms

PHASE 3: Peaking

Squat	Main work: 3x3 @ 85%	Main work: 3x2 @ 90%	Main work: 3x1 @ 95%
	Supplemental lift #1: Reverse band squat 3x3 @ 95%	Supplemental lift #1: Reverse band squat 2x3 @ 100%	Supplemental lift #1: Reverse band squat 1x3 @ 105%

	Supplemental lift #2 Pause Squat 2x3 @ 75% Accessory work to target weakness/for symmetry	Supplemental lift #2: Pause Squat 2x2 @ 80% Accessory work to target weakness/for symmetry	Supplemental lift #2: Pause Squat 2x1 @85% Accessory work to target weakness/for symmetry
Bench Press	Main work: 3x3 @ 85% Supplemental lift #1: Slingshot bench 3x3 @ 95% Supplemental lift #2: 3-second pause bench 2x3 @ 75% Accessory work to target weakness/for symmetry	Main work: 3x2 @ 90% Supplemental lift #1: Slingshot bench 2x3 @ 100% Supplemental lift #2: 3-second pause bench 2x2 @ 80% Accessory work to target weakness/for symmetry	Main work: 3x1 @ 95% Supplemental lift #1: Slingshot bench 1x3 @ 105% Supplemental lift #2: 3-second pause bench 2x1 @85% Accessory work to target weakness/for symmetry
Deadlift	Main work: 3x3 @ 85% Supplemental lift #1: 4-inch block pull 3x3 @ 95% Supplemental lift #2: Deficit deadlift 2x3 @ 75% Accessory work to target weakness/for symmetry	Main work: 3x2 @ 90% Supplemental lift #1: 4-inch block pull 2x3 @ 100% Supplemental lift #2: Deficit deadlift 2x2 @ 80% Accessory work to target weakness/for symmetry	Main work: 3x1 @ 95% Supplemental lift #1: 4-inch block pull 1x3 @ 105% Supplemental lift #2: Deficit deadlift 2x1 @85% Accessory work to target weakness/for symmetry
Military Press	Main work: 3x3 @ 85% Accessory work for the shoulders, traps, and arms	Main work: 3x2 @ 90% Accessory work for the shoulders, traps, and arms	Main work: 3x1 @ 95% Accessory work for the shoulders, traps, and arms

Here, hypothetical lifter added an additional supplemental lift for more volume and to attack more areas of the competition lift, using the formula of 10% above the working percentage for overload lifts and 10% lower for extended range of motion or pause lifts. Hypothetical lifter can play with this cycle with many different variations in terms of block length and complexity. Hypothetical lifter can then also swap out the supplemental lifts for subsequent cycles. This type of training can be successful for a long period of time. Note that hypothetical lifter may want to insert a secondary bench workout on the military press day using the heavy day/light day formula discussed above.

Advanced training for hypothetical lifter

Suppose that after several years or so of this kind of intermediate block periodization, hypothetical lifter is now ready to move on to advanced training. At this point, hypothetical lifter is the role model of the community, and is asked to speak at commencement ceremonies and to the kids at the local community center. Everyone wants to know the big secret. Hypothetical lifter is gracious yet amused knowing that all he has done is rely on the basic principles discussed in this text, and has followed the systematic plan outlined above. Being an advanced lifter, hypothetical lifter is now looking at year-long macro cycles which culminate in a realization event. Hypothetical lifter then designs the following advanced block to keep the gains coming:

Squat	Bench Press	Deadlift	Military/Bench
January-March (3 months)	January-March (3 months)	January-March (3 months)	January-March (3 months)
Main lift: close-stance squat with the safety squat bar to build the quads and upper	Main lift: Neutral grip bench to build the triceps and to drill lat engagement,	Main lift: Conventional deadlift (assuming a sumo deadlifter, i.e. weaker stance),	Main Lift: Seated Military Press, hypertrophy rep

back, hypertrophy rep range of 6-12 reps Supplemental lift: Paused squat to drill the technique with less intensity Accessory work as needed	hypertrophy rep range of 6-12 reps Supplemental lift: Cambered Bar Spoto Press to continue drilling control and reversal strength Accessory work	hypertrophy rep range of 6-12 reps Supplemental lift: Sumo deadlift (i.e. stronger stance) double pause deadlifts (pause off the floor and at the knee) Accessory work	range of 6-12 reps Supplemental lift: weighted dips Accessory work
April-June (3 months) Main lift: close-stance squat with the safety squat bar to build the quads and upper back, strength rep range 4-6 reps, hypothetical lifter then tests at the end of this cycle and logs down his record for next time Supplemental lift: Box squats to build the hips in the conventional squat Accessories as needed	April-June (3 months) Main lift: Neutral grip bench to build the triceps and to drill lat engagement, strength rep range 4-6 reps, hypothetical lifter then tests at the end of this cycle and logs down his record for next time Supplemental lift: Straight bar Spoto press with 2-second pause Accessory work	April-June (3 months) Main lift: Conventional deadlift (assuming a sumo deadlifter, i.e. weaker stance), strength rep range 4-6 reps, hypothetical lifter then tests at the end of this cycle and logs down his record for next time. Supplemental lift: Pause sumo deadlift (i.e. stronger stance) (this time one pause where lifter is weakest) Accessory work	April-June (3 months) Main Lift: Seated Military Press, strength rep range 4-6 reps, hypothetical lifter then tests at the end of this cycle and logs down his record for next time Supplemental lift: standing DB shoulder press Accessory work
July-September (3 months)	July-September (3 months)	July-September (3 months)	July-September (3 months)

Front Squat (hypertrophy 6 weeks and strength 6 weeks) Speed Squat (70-85%) for good speed and technique Accessory work	Buffalo bar bench (hypertrophy 6 weeks and strength 6 weeks) Speed Bench (70-85%) for good speed and technique Accessory work	Sumo small deficit deadlift (i.e. stronger stance from a small deficit) (hypertrophy 6 weeks and strength 6 weeks) Weaker stance speed deadlift, 70-85% for good speed and technique Accessory work	Standing military press, full 12 week hypertrophy and strength cycle, new record Accessory work
October-December Return to conventional squat, hypertrophy 3 weeks, strength 6 weeks, peaking 3 weeks New max is established.	October-December Return to the conventional bench press, hypertrophy 3 weeks, strength 6 weeks, peaking 3 weeks New max is established.	October-December Stronger stance deadlift from the floor, hypertrophy 3 weeks, strength 6 weeks, peaking 3 weeks New max is established.	October-December Bench press (light day 2x10-20 reps Seated Military Press Accessory work

Let's quickly dissect what we did here. First, hypothetical lifter switched the main lift from the traditional squat, bench, and deadlift to an exercise variation to strengthen weak muscle groups. For the squat, hypothetical lifter identified the quads as an area of concern, and began by using the close stance safety bar squat to address that concern. Because close stance safety bar squat is quite similar to the traditional back squat, improving that lift will improve the squat, without having to train the squat. The load will also end up being lighter, saving hypothetical lifter's nervous system while still allowing him to improve (i.e. modulating intensity). Hypothetical lifter uses the pause squat as the supplemental lift mostly for continuity in the movement pattern of the traditional squat, meaning that since hypothetical lifter is an early advanced trainee, he or she does not want to completely eliminate the movement pattern. The pause squat is a good choice because really challenging the pause will allow good work to be done with less weight, again sparing the nervous system. The same is true with the box squat selection in the second quarter of the year. In the third quarter of the year, hypothetical lifter switches the main lift to the front squat, which again addresses the quads but is more specific to the barbell back squat. Hypothetical lifter then begins to rev up the back squat with speed work. Finally, in the last quarter of the year, hypothetical lifter, having addressed his weaknesses, returns to the traditional back squat for an attempt at a new record. As the year progressed, notice that hypothetical lifter started with a less specific exercise and gradually moved toward more specific exercise as it became closer to returning to the competition lift. As you can see above, this was done for each lift.

Strength training is made up of both large and small waves executed over a set period of time. The complexity of the waves increase as the lifter attains greater and greater mastery of the movements. We start by just increasing weight each week, keeping all other variables stable. When we can't add weight each week, we then use larger waves to get the desired training effect (i.e. repeating 3-4 week blocks). When we can no longer do that, then we break it into longer blocks, 12 weeks or so. Then we add heavy and light days to get more volume. Then we begin to organize blocks over the longer term, as little as 16 weeks and as great as a year. Eventually, we will program training over a year's time or longer. When we make a yearly plan, the example of which is above, we don't plan all the specifics, all the sets and reps and exercises we will use. Instead, we program the blocks from 50,000 feet, then we can work out the minute details as we go, with an eye towards identifying and addressing weaknesses. While there is variation on the day-to-day level, the principles are always the same. Keep progressing in weight by raising your working max, use your most recent test numbers, this establishes a new, higher baseline every time. Keep moving from higher volume and lower intensity to high intensity and lower volume. As long as you have that in mind, and as long as you structure your workouts as I have explained, the reality is you can't really go wrong.

I hope that from this chapter you have gotten a feel as to how this operates. This chapter was designed just to provide you with an example of how a lifter starting from the foundations level can use the principles we have discussed to continue to progress from the earlies days of training to possibly elite levels, depending on the desire of the athlete and the length of the athlete's career.

Chapter 9: Warm-up and mobility

Doing a short, active warm-up is extremely important for your performance. I remember as a younger lifter, I would walk right from the street to the barbell. I also see a large number of people doing it today. This is a very poor idea. If you intend to maximize your performance, it is advisable to take about ten minutes to get your body and mind ready for the workout.

The goals of the warm up are to increase body temperature and warm up the muscles that will be involved in the training session by stretching and activating them dynamically. Research has revealed that a well-designed, dynamic warm-up can increase blood flow in the muscles, improve muscular strength and power, and lead to faster muscle contraction in the agonist and antagonist muscle groups (i.e. the muscle performing the lift, agonist, and the muscle stabilizing to allow the agonist to work, the antagonist).

In terms of mentality, the warm-up is the time to transition in your mind from the cares and concerns of the outside world to being completely mentally present for the task at hand. If you have ever practiced yoga, or any real discipline, there is an emphasis on being completely present during your practice. In yoga, your focus is only on your mat and moving through your movements and/or flow. The gym should be respected in the same way. The gym is a workplace for practitioners of their craft, it is not a social club or a time to discuss your weekend plans. Sharpen your focus for the work to come, and approach the barbell with a clear mind, focusing on each individual rep.

There are a few modalities that I like to use depending on the day:

1) Foam rolling

- Upper back
- Lats

- Thoracic spine

- Glutes

- Hamstrings

- Quads

- groin

- calves

2) Active warm-up drills for the hips

- X-band walks or Hip Circle walks (forward and backward)

- Side shuffle with X-band or Hip Circle

- bodyweight squats with Hip Circle or hip band

- kneeling lateral hip raises and hip circles, straight leg hip raises

- 90-degree hip stretch

- cradle walks

- Walking gate swings

- Standing hip swings

- Spiderman stretch

3) Groin

- lateral lunge

- half kneeling groin mobilizations

- Standing clam shells (can add a light band)

4) Glutes

- standard glute bridges (can add hip band or Hip Circle)

- single leg glute bridges

- Kneeling/standing hip circle or hip band kickbacks

5) Hamstrings

- walking toe touches

- banded good mornings

- walking Frankenstein kicks

- standing kicks/swings

- Inchworm walks

- lunge walks

6) Low back

- Banded good mornings

- light hyperextensions or reverse hypers

- "Superman" holds

7) Lats/back

- Banded rows and pullovers

- Three-point thoracic extension

- banded lat stretch

- cable/band pullovers

8) Shoulders

- "no monies" (can also be banded)

- band pull aparts

- Overhead band pull aparts

- band external/internal rotation

- face pull to external rotation (kneeling or standing, cable or band)

- Banded arm circles (forward and backward)

- wall slides

- banded, front-facing wall slides

- banded hand crawls

9) Full body warm-ups

- bear crawls

- spider crawls

Generally speaking, we will select a handful of exercises to perform prior to each workout, which will generally last around ten minutes. Your warm-up is exactly that, a chance to prepare the body for the real work. These are not working sets or designed to create fatigue, leave that to the actual lifts. I will share my template as to how I generally warm up before each of the main lifts.

Exercise	Warm-up template
Squat	Focuses for me: hips, groin, and hamstrings Foam rolling: - back: upper to lower (10 reps) - thoracic extension on foam roller (10 reps) - upper hamstring (10-20 reps per leg) - full hamstring (10-20 reps per leg) - upper groin (10-20 reps per leg) - full groin to knee (10-20 reps per leg) Dynamic warm-up: - Hip Circle or X-band walks 3x10 steps/leg - side shuffle with Hip Circle or X-band 3x10 steps/leg - Hip circle squat 1x10-20 - side lunge with groin stretch 10 steps/side

	- Walking Frankenstein kicks 10/leg - kneeling lateral hip raise with hip circle 10 of each/leg - walking lunge 10/leg - half-kneeling groin mobs 10-20/leg - band pull aparts and arm circles (20 and 20)
Bench Press	Focus: lats and shoulders Foam rolling: - back: upper to lower (10 reps) - thoracic extension on foam roller (10 reps) - lats (10/side) - upper hamstring (10-20 reps per leg) - full hamstring (10-20 reps per leg) - upper groin (10-20 reps per leg) - full groin to knee (10-20 reps per leg) Dynamic warm-up: - Hip Circle or X-band walks 3x10 steps/leg - side shuffle with Hip Circle or X-band 3x10 steps/leg - band or cable pullovers 3x10-20 - Band palms down row (3x10-20) - Band pull aparts (3x20-30) - Overhead band pull aparts (3x10-12)
Deadlift	Focuses for me: hips, groin, and hamstrings Foam rolling: - back: upper to lower (10 reps) - thoracic extension on foam roller (10 reps) - upper hamstring (10-20 reps per leg) - full hamstring (10-20 reps per leg) - upper groin (10-20 reps per leg) - full groin to knee (10-20 reps per leg)

	Dynamic warm-up: • Hip Circle or X-band walks 3x10 steps/leg • side shuffle with Hip Circle or X-band 3x10 steps/leg • Hip circle squat 1x10-20 • side lunge with groin stretch 10 steps/side • Walking Frankenstein kicks 10/leg • kneeling lateral hip raise with hip circle 10 of each/leg • walking lunge 10/leg • half-kneeling groin mobs 10-20/leg • kneeling rocking stretch 3x10-12 • band pull aparts and arm circles (20 and 20)
Military Press	Focus: lats and shoulders Foam rolling: • back: upper to lower (10 reps) • thoracic extension on foam roller (10 reps) • lats (10/side) • upper hamstring (10-20 reps per leg) • full hamstring (10-20 reps per leg) • upper groin (10-20 reps per leg) • full groin to knee (10-20 reps per leg) Dynamic warm-up: • Hip Circle or X-band walks 3x10 steps/leg • side shuffle with Hip Circle or X-band 3x10 steps/leg • band or cable pullovers 3x10-20 • Band palms down row (3x10-20) • Band pull aparts (3x20-30) • Overhead band pull aparts (3x10-12) • Band "no monies" (10) • Band internal/external rotation (10 each)

Additional mobility work can be performed in separate workouts either on off days or later/earlier in the day on workout days. Any one of the above can be repeated, or in separate workouts separate from your actual workout, you can incorporate other techniques such as PNF (proprioceptive neuromuscular facilitation) stretching with a partner or with bands. This is up to you depending on your individual needs. When it comes to the warm-up, however, get in, get a sweat, and get going.

Chapter 10: Deload

A deload or unloading workout/microcycle is a technique in which you plan a light workout or week of training to allow the body to recover and adapt to the heavier training, and "supercompensate" by reaching a new level of fitness. This is essentially the general adaptation cycle that we discussed at greater length, above. After completing a hard training session, our performance will actually decrease for a period of time (known as the "alarm phase"). For example, if you were planning to attempt a new one rep max squat, you would not want to do a hard squat workout the day before. Why? Because the workout on the day before the max attempt would, temporarily, decrease your ability to perform on the squat, and ultimately sabotage your efforts at a new one rep max the following day. However, once a training session is over, the body will begin the compensation phase (i.e. a return to homeostasis). If the training is properly programmed and nutrition and rest are proper, the body will ultimately rebound into a state of supercompensation, meaning that the athlete has established a new, increased level of homeostasis. Two things can sabotage this. The first is overtraining, such that the training is so intense and so frequent that the athlete never recovers and is unable to reach supercompensation. The second is detraining, meaning that the athlete had achieved a state of supercompensation but because there was too long of a span between the supercompensation and the next training session, the athlete's new level of homeostasis regressed.

The idea here is not to make this a textbook, but to help you put the concept of deloading in its proper place. Key times to deload are as follows:

1) **At the end of a peaking block before establishing a new one-rep max.** The rationale here should be clear. By using a targeted unloading week before our highest performance is required, we allow the body to fully recover to take advantage of the

supercompensation effect. People sometimes call this "delayed transformation." Less advanced athletes may need only a few days for optimal performance, whereas very advanced athletes may need up to three weeks. This has to do with the total volume load. An advanced lifter has a significantly higher volume load than a beginner or intermediate lifter, and as a result is carrying more fatigue. The idea of the deload is to shed the fatigue to allow for optimal performance. To graft this onto our categories above, a beginner lifter may want to take 2-3 days off from the gym before the one-rep max attempt at the end of the beginner cycle. An intermediate lifter will generally take one week before a realization event, and may want to incorporate one day of light technique work for 3-5 sets of 1-5 reps between 30-50% during that week. An advanced trainee may use 2-3 weeks with a "taper" (i.e. a gradual decline in volume load) which leads to a deload week of one day of light technique work for 3-5 sets of 1-5 reps between 30-50% the week before the realization event.

2) **After a new one-rep max attempt is taken.** After year peak and your establishing of a new one rep max (or attempt to establish a new one-rep max), you should take time away to allow the body to recover from that event before starting a new training block. This too depends on how advanced the lifter is. The beginner lifter may want to take 3-4 days before switching to intermediate programming. An intermediate trainee may want to take a week. An advanced trainee may want to take two weeks or more. During this period, light GPP work can be done.

3) **At strategic times during the training cycle.**

    a. **Beginner**

For a beginner lifter, or someone who is new to the weight room, I see very little need for planned deloads. At that point, the lifter is still learning the movements. Chances are technique is not yet optimal so the trainee is using overall lighter loads. However, some good ideas would be to plan a deload during a particularly oppressive week at work or school (i.e. during finals week), or during the week of a planned vacation. At the end of the day, stress is stress. Stress from your job or from school will add to the cumulative stress you accrue in the weight room. So if you know in advance that there is a bad week coming up, it is sensible to plan a deload where you still train your prescribed days, but at a lighter load (i.e. 50-60% of your calculated max). If you are a lunatic like me, vacation does not stop you from finding a barbell. But I understand some people would prefer that the majority of their vacation is outside the gym, and sometimes people travel to destinations with very minimal resort equipment. In that case, train for fun, do something useful, and call it a day. Be resourceful, use what you have.

A beginner should also plan a short deload before the one-rep max attempt at the end of the beginner cycle. For most people, 3-4 days will be plenty. I would say no more than a week barring exceptional circumstances. A similar break should be taken after the one-rep max attempt.

b. Intermediate

A lower intermediate lifter using the three-week wave program can generally deload as often as every six weeks, or may choose to go 9-12 weeks before deloading. As a general rule, a newer intermediate lifter can probably go as far as 12 weeks before taking a delaod. As the lifter becomes more advanced (and thus starts working with heavier loads), deloads can gradually become more frequent to every six weeks. In certain circumstances, the lifter may want to incorporate a deload after each three-week block toward the end of the cycle to complete as many cycles as possible.

As touched on above, life circumstances may necessitate the taking of a deload week or workout. Further, if a lifter is feeling particularly beaten and worn down, it may be wise to plan an unloading week and return to program. A deload period of approximately a week should be used before and after maximal attempts.

c. Advanced

An advanced lifter will follow the same general parameters as the intermediate lifter. A good time to deload would be between cycles of training. These can be planned out within the lifter's yearly plan (i.e. macrocycle). The advanced trainee will also have a greater ability to go by feel and know when a deload cycle is required. A taper and deload should be taken before maximal attempts. A deload period should be taken after the realization event. As discussed above, life events are always relevant in determining planned deload cycles.

Part 3: Adamantine Nutrition

Chapter 11: Fueling the Body

The number one commandment when it comes to nutrition is that you must eat to fuel your performance. You will notice at the outset that the title of this chapter is not "diet" or "nutrition," it is entitled fueling the body. From this day forward, you will think of eating in terms of providing your body with the resources it needs to succeed in the weight room and to become stronger.

At the outset, for someone beginning his or her fitness journey, nutrition can be a daunting concept. That is because there have been thousands of books written on diet, and manty times they will contain contradictory information. Here is the real truth: diet, like training, is all about strong fundamentals and basic steps applied consistently over time (surprise!). This is not sexy; there is no magic. If you want to be in shape and be reasonably lean, healthy, and have muscle, you need to eat quality food. Be very wary of anyone who tells you otherwise. If you follow any competitive bodybuilder on his or her way to a competition, you will see they are eating fish and meat, vegetables, and quality carbs. They are not stuffing their face with cakes and candies. That is not to say that there is no room for moderation, it is just to say that you must apply consistency over time.

Let's start by reviewing some foundation principles with regard to diet. The first thing we need to review are macronutrients. Macronutrients are nutrients that we are required to consume a large amount of on a day-to-day basis to live. They give us the energy our body needs to function. There are three macronutrients: protein, lipids (fat), and carbs. Protein is the most highly marketed supplement and most referenced macronutient when it comes to muscle gain. Protein is similar to carbs and fats, except protein contains nitrogen (i.e. amino acids). Amino acids are further divided into essential (i.e. EAAs) and non-essential amino acids. A non-essential amino acid is one that is synthesized in the body, an essential one is on we must consume in our diet. Skeletal muscle is composed of protein. Therefore, it is important that we consume sufficient amounts of protein for the growth and maintenance of skeletal muscle. Foods such as meats, fish, eggs, and dairy products are generally known as "high-quality proteins," proteins of "high biological value" or "complete proteins" because they contain amino acids needed by the body (i.e. essential amino acids). This is why the above-referenced foods tend to be the staples of bodybuilding and performance athlete diets. For people in athletic populations (i.e. people who train to enhance their bodies in some way or for a certain task beyond mere survival and day-to-day tasks), the research generally suggests about 1.7 grams of protein per kilogram of bodyweight. Guys at the gym usually use the rule of thumb of one gram of protein per pound of bodyweight.

As for carbohydrates, they provide an energy source. Consuming carbohydrates increases muscle and liver glycogen stores, which you can think about like gas tank. It is stored by the body to be used in our daily locomotion and survival, as well as for training. Carbohydrate sources are vast but most commonly include oats and grains, bread (or similar common products such as cereal, granola bars, etc.), pasta, fruits, potatoes, rice, quinoa, among others. Drilling down a little further, carbohydrates can either be "fast" or "slow." This refers to the famous "glycemic index," which essentially seeks to measure how long (and how high) a particular carbohydrate raises blood glucose. A rapid raise in blood glucose is also associated with a spike in insulin, which can be good or bad depending on the time. Sources such as brown rice, whole grain/whole wheat breads, sweet potato, oats and wheat germ, and quinoa are examples of "slower" carbs. Things like white bread, cakes and candies, waffles, white potatoes, bagels and white rice are "faster" and tend to be more highly glycemic. Generally speaking, athletes who are engaging in the type of workouts described herein would benefit from approximately six grams of carbohydrate per kilogram of bodyweight. This can vary depending on how fat or skinny you happen to be.

The last main macronutrient is lipids/fat. Fat is the most dense macronutrient, providing 9 calories per gram of bodyweight. Fats, like carbs, are an energy source for the body. Examples of fats include things such as nuts (and peanut butter), oils (vegetable, canola, coconut, etc.), fish such as salmon, avocado, bacon, etc. Fat usually makes up the smallest portion of the daily diet because of its high caloric density and because of the ease in which it can be stored as body fat. However, there are essential fats that are positive for us, these are your omega-3 and omega-6 fats. Things like salmon, nuts, and avocado are good sources. It is also why you see supplements containing fish oil and flax seed oil. On the other hand, saturated fats generally can only be used as energy or stored as fat (i.e. butter, cream, fatty meats, etc.). Excess consumption of saturated fat also is responsible for raising cholesterol levels. With that said, diets that are extremely low in fat tend to have the adverse effect of reducing testosterone and hindering the body's performance. Generally, fat will account for about 20% of the daily calorie consumption when operating under a general balanced diet.

After macronutrients, there are micronutrients. Micronutrients are required in smaller amounts than macronutrients. The two basic types of micronutrients are vitamins and minerals, which are also obtained from a balanced and healthy diet. Some people rely on multivitamins to ensure that they are meeting their daily micronutrient requirements.

That is the general backdrop, now, as I said before, I endeavor to make the nutrition portion of this book as simple as possible. Here are the guiding principles I suggest:

1. **The ordinary person does not need to count anything.** This probably sounds like absolute blasphemy to many, if not all, of the diet gurus who have written volumes on counting calories, counting macros, weighing food and portions, etc. The truth is for people who are busy, who have families, businesses, school, obligations, it adds tremendous stress and is really just not necessary. Instead of counting, I would recommend making adjustments depending on goal and body type, discussed in more detail below.

2. **Every meal you eat should include a quality, complete protein source.** We discussed complete proteins above. I suggest making it a habit to eat quality protein at each meal. This is not as hard as it sounds. Eggs and/or egg whites in the morning. Chicken, 90+% lean ground turkey, 90+% lean beef, fish (i.e. Cod, Tilapia, etc.), or lean steak during the day for your afternoon and evening meals. Your quality protein should take precedence and be consumed first and consumed thoroughly.

3. **Eat frequently enough such that you are never hungry.** This is an important rule and the main reason why we don't have to count anything, and that's because your body is usually pretty good at telling you things. If, while training in the way I have outlined above, you are regularly feeling hungry, that is your body telling you that you aren't consuming enough to fuel your performance. At that point, you must plan to eat more. For those of you who are stressed about this, it's generally a good idea to eat every 2-4 hours. A normal day for me would be breakfast before work at around 7 a.m. I usually bring a shake or protein bar for my travels to snack on, first lunch at 11 a.m., second lunch between 1 and 2 p.m., next meal between 4-5 p.m., and then dinner around 8-9 p.m.

I have found success with this general schedule. This is ignoring peri-workout nutrition for now.

4. **Fruits and vegetables are not wrong to eat, I don't care what they tell you.** Unless you have some sort of allergy or medical issue, you should never be concerned about consuming fruits and vegetables. Vegetables are good because they tend to be a rich source of vitamins and minerals (i.e. micronutrients), as well as fiber and antioxidants in many cases. It is good to get into the habit of consuming vegetables throughout the day. Fruits are also good, and will also provide you with the vitamins and minerals you need. Many are lower on the glycemic index than most of our common American carbohydrate sources. But even if they aren't, eating a serving of fruits or vegetables is not going to be so tremendously dense that substantial fat storage will occur. In sum, fruits and vegetables are good for you, eat them.

5. **Consume your carbs from high-quality sources rather than junk.** The majority of your carbohydrate intake should come from fruits and vegetables, oats, sweet potato, brown rice and/or quinoa. During periods of intense training especially, whole wheat pasta and quality whole grain breads can be relied upon. There are also some cool products out there like Kodiak Cakes which are high protein, whole grain muffins and flapjacks. Products like that can be used especially pre- and post- workout, such that you are actually consuming some quality ingredients while taking advantage of the fast-acting carbs and associated insulin spike. White rice and white potatoes, things of that nature, are also good around workouts. Personally, I like to have a little white rice before workouts or after workouts when possible. You should avoid routinely consuming carbohydrates from junk sources: cakes, candies, pies, high-sugar cereals, chips, cookies,

and drinking 20 beers with your weak, average friends. That's all garbage. Get in the habit of avoiding things that make you average.

6. **Drinks should not be more than zero calories, unless it's a shake.** I have found that as a general rule, anything that is consumed as a drink with calories is probably garbage. Soda, high calorie energy drinks, high-sugar teas, soft drinks, etc., is a huge part of what is making America obese. Like smoking, these drinks are all detriment for no reward. Drink mostly water. Coffee and tea are good if you are inclined to drink either for luxury or for a pick me up, but don't load it up with cream and sugar. Suck it up. If you want to use a little reduced fat milk or half and half, and a little Truvia or Stevia, fine. The only permissible time you should be drinking beverages with calories is when you are preparing a protein shake. As a snack or in between meals, you may want to prepare a shake with some reduced (or no) fat milk, whey protein, peanut butter, oats, fruits and vegetables, etc. This is a good way to get more quality calories in and also a good way to get more vegetables in if you dislike eating vegetables.

7. **Prepare to win.** When I was young, my wrestling coach gave us a poster with the famous Muhammad Ali quote: "The fight is won or lost far away from the witnesses, behind the lines, in the gym, and out there on the road; long before I dance under those lights." Over that famous quote, in bold, was the words **"PREPARE TO WIN."** I carried that poster with me through my entire life, because it is true for everything, and success in the gym is no different. Your days of not planning your meals and not being consistent with your nutrition are over. Remember, part time athletes get part time results. Everyone is busy, everyone has obligations. Suck it up. Everywhere you go, work, school, family parties and get-togethers, you will have a plan for your meals. As we discussed above:

complete protein source, vegetables and/or fruit, quality carb. If you will be in a meeting, an exam, or some event that you know will take a great deal of time, prepare a shake that you can sip on throughout the event, that way you don't lose out, then afterwards consume a meal when you can. Prep in advance, cook everything on one day, I don't care, just get it done.

You now know everything you need to know about fueling the body. The last thing I would like to do before we move on is provide you with some templates depending on body type, and some diet suggestions for each:

TYPE 1: Skinny and underweight

If you are skinny and underweight, and lack muscle mass, unless you have a medical condition, you need to make eating, and eating big, a top priority. Having worked with many high school athletes, many of them desire to add substantial muscle, but woefully under-eat. I would ask them, upon arriving for the training session, the same question: What have you eaten today? For the first few weeks, I received the same blank stare and answer. But being fortunate to work with some very highly-motivated kids, after the first few days they got the hint, and had a good answer. From there, they began to add substantial muscle because they began to realize the importance of eating, and more importantly of not making excuses. Every once in a while, you will get a stubborn, 130-pound kid who will complain about losing his "abs," at which point you simply explain that he should look like he lifts to the casual observer on the street, and that once you fix that problem, you can move on to honing the abs.

If you are very skinny, that is a good place to be, because you can open up the diet more and really get a lot of calories. If you are training as I have prescribed, you can eat a heck of a lot and add a substantial amount of muscle with limited fat gain. Long story short, you need to eat.

TYPE 2: Overweight to Substantially Overweight

If you are starting out with a substantial amount of body fat, you will want to focus on eating high protein with moderate to slightly below moderate amounts of carbohydrate and fat. This will help you, in combination with the training, to lose fat while maintaining and building muscle mass. One tweak I would suggest for someone who is overweight would be to consume only a complete protein and vegetables wherever possible. For any meals other than pre- and post-workout meals, I would suggest that fruit be the only carb source. Pre- and post-training, quality carbs such as oats or rice may be consumed. Follow this patter until you significantly decrease your body fat, then you may slowly begin adding more carbs, as needed.

TYPE 3: Moderate or athletic build

Some of you may be starting during or after playing competitive sports or with a decent background of general resistance training, and as a result already have a fairly muscular or athletic build. In that case, the diet is simple. Be sure to eat every 2-3 hours with a lean, complete protein, a quality carb of choice, and vegetables. Make it a point to hit your protein macros. No reason to re-invent the wheel.

Chapter 12: Navigating Supplements

There is an old saying to "be wary of strangers bearing gifts," this is sound advice when venturing into the world of sports supplements and dietary supplements. It is no surprise that the sports supplement industry has become over a billion-dollar industry, because it relies on the same underlying narrative that every scam and trick has relied on since the beginning of time: I will give you something of great value, and it will cost you nothing. That line of thinking is antithetical to the Adamantine Strength mindset. We know that nothing of value comes without hard work, dedication, and sound fundamentals. Think I'm lying or being a curmudgeon? Go to your local library and look through the fitness magazines from two to three years ago, five years ago, and look at all the "groundbreaking" supplements that were being advertised that we could not live without. Now go to that magazines most recent issue, or to your local health store and stroll the aisles, and see how many are still on the market today. You will see that it is alarmingly few. There have been numerous lawsuits against companies that manufacture dietary supplements because they do not do what they claim to do, because they are overtly harmful, and because of misrepresentation and deceptive marketing practices. Just because something is sold at a local health store does not mean that it is "safe" or desirable. You, the athlete, have the responsibility to know what you are putting into your body.

With that general warning aside, I am not anti-supplement. I just believe that they should be put in their proper place. The first rule is that there is no supplement or drug in the world that will give us results for nothing. If you do not train hard, no supplement will profit you. If your diet is horrible, no supplement will profit you. Supplements can be the proverbial icing on the cake when the other pillars of training, nutrition, and recovery are in place.

Supplements can serve one of two functions: 1) they can be used for convenience; and 2) they can be used to bring something to your diet that you do not ordinarily get from food.

First, as to convenience, I indicated before that almost everyone has a busy life. Whether you are in school, working, being a parent, etc., everyone has a lot of responsibility. One supplement that can be very good for convenience is a good, quality whey protein/whey protein isolate. Whey protein is perhaps the most known and most marketed sports supplement, and for pretty good reason. Whey is one of the two main sources of protein in milk (the other is casein), and a very high-quality protein at that. Whey protein is good because it both contains all twenty amino acids, and has high levels of the amino acids most noteworthy for performance and muscle gain, to wit leucine, isoleucine, valine, and glutamine (a lot of times these amino acids will be marketed independently as supplements or part of a "BCAA" product, but all will be contained in your whey). The research has generally been favorable in regards to consumption of whey protein, especially before and after training. Some people advocate adding some fast-acting carbs to create an insulin spike which they feel improves absorption into the muscles. I'm cool with that if that's something you want to do.

I also generally think having a good whey protein powder is good for a quality snack if you are on the go. For example, long meetings or classes, etc., you may want to plan by making a shake with whey protein to keep your muscles fed through the long period of not eating. You may also want to add some reduced-fat milk and other things such as natural peanut butter, oats, and/or fruit/vegetables to get more calories. These can help hold you over between meals. Again, no supplement is mandatory. You can do perfectly fine without any supplements at all. I make the suggestion for people who are interested and for whom it may be useful.

Building off of the above, because many people have very busy schedules, a lot of times they train early in the morning or late at night. Therefore, you may want to use a little caffeine before workouts to assist with focus and performance. This does not require tremendous explanation, many people drink beverages such as coffee and energy drinks while at work or at school to improve focus. You may want to have a cup of coffee before a workout or your beverage of choice (that is zero calories). If neither of those are agreeable to you, you can get caffeine pills at your local health store or probably at your local pharmacy for minimal cost. If you are sensitive to caffeine or it is not agreeable to you, there is no need to force it. It will not make or break your gains.

The last supplement that can be used for convenience is creatine monohydrate. Other than whey protein, creatine monohydrate is perhaps the most marketed and talked about sports supplement. To understand the true effects of creatine, we need just a little boring science. The kind of training we are engaging in as described above can be characterized as short-term, high intensity exercise. We are lifting relatively heavy weights for a relatively short period of time, unlike, for example, a marathon runner that must maintain a consistent stream of energy over a long duration. The reason this is significant is because your body has different means of producing energy depending on the type of training you are doing. For us, the prime producer of energy will be the phosphagen system, which produces something called adenosine triphosphate (ATP) for energy (i.e. to contract muscle fibers). When ATP is used for energy, it is broken town to adenosine diphosphate. The phosphagen system replenishes ATP by catalyzing ADP with creatine phosphate, which is stored in relatively small quantities in the muscle, to produce more ATP and thus perform better for longer. From the above explanation, you can begin to see the rub. Researchers then sought to insert more creatine, by oral supplementation, to see if the body could then produce more

ATP and thus increase performance. This increase in ATP then leads to greater strength and muscle gains. Creatine monohydrate converts to creatine phosphate when ingested, and that is why it is popular.

Now this is no reason to go crazy and run down the street to spend your week's pay stocking up on creatine. Remember, we are talking about the icing on the cake here, just one little thing to give us a slight edge when everything else is in place. No supplement will take you from zero to hero, and if you do not use any supplements, you will be more than fine so long as you train and eat properly. If you do come to the point where you wish to use creatine monohydrate as a dietary supplement, just do yourself a favor and get a simple creatine monohydrate supplement, your gains will be the same and you will save money.

The second classification of supplements are those which add something to your diet that you would not otherwise get a sufficient quantity of in your daily diet. For me, the big supplement that fits into this category is a good fish oil supplement. The truth is that I am just not a big fish eater. I know it's good for me, but I know that if the choice is between fish and something like chicken or beef, I am probably always going to choose the latter. But, fish has a lot of good qualities that I might not be getting otherwise. Enter a fish oil supplement. A good fish oil supplement will provide you with a sufficient quantity of EPA and DHA, essential fatty acids which are positive for both heart and brain health. It's been generally accepted that taking a good fish oil supplement is a pretty good idea for various reasons. Even if you do eat fish from time to time, chances are you still are not getting enough of these essential fatty acids. So fish oil is a prime example of a supplement that can be used to include something in your diet you would not otherwise get.

That's about it for supplements. None of them are 100% necessary, and you will do fine without them so long as you eat a healthy and balanced diet and hit your protein macros. But if you would like to delve into that world, you have my advice.

Part 4: Adamantine Mindset

Chapter 13: Two Wolves

An old Cherokee is teaching his grandson about life. "A fight is going on inside me," he said to the boy.

"It is a terrible fight and it is between two wolves. One is evil – he is anger, envy, sorrow, regret, greed, arrogance, self-pity, guilt, resentment, inferiority, lies, false pride, superiority, and ego." He continued, "The other is good – he is joy, peace, love, hope, serenity, humility, kindness, benevolence, empathy, generosity, truth, compassion, and faith. The same fight is going on inside you – and inside every other person, too."

The grandson thought about it for a minute and then asked his grandfather, "Which wolf will win?"

The old Cherokee simply replied, "The one you feed."

I love this old Cherokee parable because it conceptualizes very succinctly the tug of war that each of us face within ourselves every day. It is the tension between the comfort of mediocrity and the discomfort of progress and advancement. It is this invisible battle that is lurking behind every choice we make in our lives, which will ultimately determine the degree of success we will reach. More so than any sets or reps or discussion about exercise and nutrition, what this book really presents you with is a choice. You can choose, today, to put yourself on the path of success, to invest in yourself and your future, and to use the fruits of your labor as a harvest, not only as a reward for yourself, but to help others along the way, to pull others up with you. That is how strong communities are built, and how prosperity is won for a society. The barbell is as good a place as any to begin to win that battle. Anyone can do it, there are no start-up costs, no barriers to entry. All you need is a gym membership or an old barbell and some plates.

I love the verbiage that is used in the parable. Look closely at the characteristics of the first wolf. First, as discussed in more detail in Chapter 2, the first wolf is ego, false pride, and arrogance, or as I have more specifically defined, the unwarranted ego. The ego of this kind is usually a coping mechanism to distort reality for the psychological benefit of the individual employing it. The individual employing this strategy usually is self-conscious about himself or herself in one or more areas, and, as a defense mechanism, creates the delusion of the ego as protection. The end result of that is the 125-pound kid flexing in the gym mirror, or the kid who hits an ugly 315-pound deadlift and then considers himself ready to coach the entire gym. Everyone can see they are delusional, except them. What is particularly destructive is that this delusion prevents forward progress by preventing a rational and objective evaluation of strengths and weaknesses. The above are obvious examples, but the ego can manifest itself more subtly as the lifter advances. It could come in the form of choosing only assistance exercises that the lifter is good at, but which are overused and have reached a point of diminishing returns. Relatedly, it can come in the form of avoiding supplemental or assistance exercises that the lifter knows will help, but will also hurt the lifter's ego in the form of having to start with less weight and reps. It can be rejecting learning or seeking to understand new programming concepts or ideas that may be different than yours. This type of delusional activity tends to be contagious, and tends to permeate to all areas of life once given a foothold.

The first wolf, interestingly, is both inferiority and superiority. It is both because both are delusions. No person/lifter is superior or inferior to any other man/lifter. A man's success is determined by his ability to objectively grasp and understand certain fundamental principles and apply them. These principles, which have underscored and are the bedrock of this entire book, existed long before you or I were born, and will exist long after we die. We did not create them; we are thankful recipients. A person's success comes from understanding these principles, standing on them in his or her actions (not just in thought), and using them to bend or manipulate matter to his or her desired end, whether it be the deadlift or the combustible engine.

The rest of the characteristics of the first wolf, I think, are effects of the unwarranted ego, namely anger, sorrow, regret, envy, and resentment. Even when the proverbial first wolf has his teeth sunk in deep into our psyche, there are always cracks in the membrane. The person harboring the cherished delusion will begin to show symptoms. They will feel anger, they will cast themselves as the victim. Others' success will be a reproach to them, rather than something to be celebrated. Their lack of progress will be someone else's fault. It will be that they don't have good enough genetics, they don't have good enough supplements, good enough knee sleeves, so on and so forth. Any excuse will do, as it preserves the delusion. If I believe that I am superior and I know everything, then if I fail, it must be someone or something's fault other than mine.

The person who is adamantine strong knows that he or she can provide no quarter whatsoever to the first wolf. The recovering alcoholic knows that it only takes one taste of alcohol to spark a full relapse. The same is true here, once you let delusion creep in, you begin to pave the way to your own destruction. The adamantine strong individual feeds only the second wolf, characterized as truth, humility, and faith. He or she knows that the training must be analyzed objectively for what is working and what is not. He or she must be able to see and understand his or her strengths and weaknesses. He or she knows that one must set out to win every single rep. Rep by rep, workout by workout, mesocycle by mesocycle, macrocycle by macrocycle, competition by competition. This is how success is achieved.

The adamantine strong individual knows that acting in this way is the anomaly in today's world, and that feeding only the second wolf will be, for a time, a lonely road. That is because normal today is weak and delusional. Normal is hoping that some overpriced supplement will provide you with a shortcut, or that your next squat PR will come from some knee wrap or knee sleeve that you don't have. Normal is looking for the easy way out, the path of least resistance. Normal is comfortable in mediocrity, and seeks relative comfort for minimal exertion. It is not for normal that I write, it is for people who want to excel in life; people who are willing to embark on the long, slow journey to success. I write for people who seek to make true progress, who want to be better each day, each week, each month, each year. People who want to look down from the mountaintop and realize that they scaled the side of the mountain to get there, while others perished either for never attempting the climb or falling at some point to the top. This will not be an easy road; in fact, there will be times it will feel like a death march. One thing I do know, however, is that it will be a fruitful one. While it will require you to disappoint your weak friends when you decline to go out drinking because you have a squat workout lined up the next morning, you will rest with the assurance that you are building something, with the assurance that you will look back at the end of the year and be stronger than you were when you started it.

You must live differently, you must have an iron moral code. You must reject excuses, victimhood, and delusions, and assess your stuff with the cold ruthlessness that comes from rejecting the crutches of delusion. Look closely at any truly successful person, and you will see these principles brought to life. You will also find that any normal person would consider their life to be crazy. Take, for example, The Rock, who everyone loves, and for good reason. The guy churns out movies like hot cakes, filming for hours and hours each day, and is up and in the gym early in the morning or late at night, many times right off a plane. His schedule would put a normal man in the emergency room in a week or less. But you will never see The Rock complain, ever. In fact, he has more enthusiasm to crush legs after a flight than the common man does coming off the couch. Not to mention he willingly eats like five servings of cod a day. He is able to do this because of the principles described in this chapter, because he feeds the second wolf, and is rewarded as a result.

At the end of the day, your success or failure is up to you. From this day forward, stop talking defeat, and stop making excuses. Stick to your plan, stay the course, and suck it up when necessary. If you ever want to complain or feel sorry for yourself, just remember there is someone out there who has won with far less than you have. Build a proper foundation, and put yourself on the path of success. It is not too late. I hope to catch my reader at a young age, but if not, remember the old Chinese proverb: "The best time to plant a tree was twenty years ago, the second best time is now." When you lay the proper foundation and apply the correct principles, there is no limit to how far you can go.

Chapter 14: You Are Either In Or You Are Out, There Is No Such Thing As A Life In Between

The title of this chapter is derived from a placard that once hung in my high school gym. Let me tell you the hard truth, while I have tried to lay out for you a path to success in lifting that is as clear and concise as possible, if you have aspirations to do this at a very high level (or really just above average), it is going to take everything you have. The reality is that most of you, probably well over 90%, will not be willing to pay the price to do it. There will be times when your training will be great, times when it will be good, and times when it will be terrible. There will be peaks, there will be valleys, there will be plateaus. It is just the nature of the game. If you are in, you will succeed. If you are out, you will fail.

What does it mean to be in? Well, what it means is that every decision you make in your day must pass the following question: Does what I am about to do bring me closer to my goal? If the answer is no, you don't do it. If the answer is yes, then you do. Further, you do what you need to do to advance your goal regardless of the circumstances, whether you feel like doing it at that time or not, every day. Rain, sleet, snow, whether you have the sniffles, whether you are tired, you get it done, no excuses. Your willingness to adopt this attitude will determine your level of success.

Let's get more practical. Start with the workout itself. We said before that everything we do in the gym is one of the four main lifts, or is a supplemental or accessory lift designed to increase one of the four main lifts. First order of business is that if what you are doing in the gym does not support that goal, cut it out. I can't begin to tell you how many people I see in the gym who either 1) do not perform the main lift at all, or 2) only perform the main lift (usually not well) for 3-4 sets, which takes about 10-15 minutes, and then spend the next 45 minutes on useless exercises. I have seen people finish entire workouts before I finish my main and supplemental exercise. The point is that you should be completely mentally and physically invested in the performance of the main lift, as it is the most important thing you will do in the gym. Everything else is designed to improve the main lift. What this also means is that you have to be "in" on the system. The Scripture says you cannot serve two masters. You cannot attempt to be a cross country skier and marathon runner and also gain maximum strength and size. At a certain point, these things will interfere with one another, and prevent full growth in any discipline. The goal of this book is to help you get strong and add muscle, to look and to feel good. The method revolves around improving the main lifts and using additional exercises to attack weak points, as well as to build the supporting muscles and to maintain balance. You must completely buy in to this system.

The next element comes when you exit the gym, namely executing on the little things throughout the day to make sure you can train to your highest potential. This is where most people will fall off the wagon. The reality is that the training is the easy part of all this, the fun part. The sacrifice required to reach your goals comes outside the gym. Let's go through them:

Many of you will fail because you will not pay the price to make sure you have your meals. When I work with high school kids especially, I always ask them a question I got from Tony Gentilcore, what did you have for breakfast? The answer, 90% of the time, is nothing. Then the excuses start: "I didn't have time," "Mom didn't replenish the eggs," "I had to study," etc. For college kids, it is even worse, as most of them have a meal plan and a short order cook at the ready, and still fail to execute. Adults are the same. They rely on the excuses of work and deadlines, family, on and on. Let me address all of these by saying that no one cares, and the barbell certainly doesn't care. If you want this, you have to make the time. Audit your day, account for every minute. Get up earlier, stop binging on Netflix shows until the early hours of the morning, stop wasting your time at work or school so you can get out and do something else. Prepare your meals for the week over the weekend if it helps, have designated days where you prepare meals. If you know there is a period where you will be away from your meals, plan to bring a shake. I know it is time consuming and not pleasant to do, but to be successful, you have to get it done. There is no way you can reach your goals without adequate nutrition. It must be consistent: Day after day, week after week, year after year. Part time athletes get part time results.

Many of you will fail because you will not sleep enough. I understand that many people have busy and stressful lives, as do I. I understand there are times when you will have to work late, be up early, or both. Some things are out of your control. What I will say about this is to minimize self-inflicted wounds. 99% of people who say they don't have time to sleep are horrible time managers. I remember in law school, it was around finals time, and there were several people who correlated working hard with how many hours they sat in the law school. More than half of that time was spent taking breaks, jerking around, and draining time on something other than the task at hand. These are the same types of people who will tell you they don't have time to prepare their meals and don't have time to train. These are weak people. Strong people don't make excuses for not getting the job done. Mike O'Hearn trains every day at 4 a.m. because that's when he has time to do so. He is "in," he is willing to pay the price to reach his goals. All of this is a game of inches, doing little things right every day. By doing the little things right over and over, you eventually change your life.

If you consider yourself "busy," start by getting the junk out of your day. When you go to the gym, attack it. Don't mess around and float around talking to everyone there. You are there to get better. When you go to work or school, attack it. Do what you are supposed to do and get out. This opens up time for your nutrition and your training, and for your family.

You might be thinking that I am a hard ass or no fun. You might be right. But what I do know is that no one ever got anywhere special with vacillation and lack of direction. Many of you picked up this book because you want to be strong, you want to have muscle, you want to build something that you are proud of. And I am telling you that this is the only way I know how to do it. If you really watch anyone who is truly successful, someone who really went the distance to achieve mastery in his or her field, you will see that they say the same thing. Ed Coan didn't deadlift 900 pounds by accident, and Ronnie Coleman didn't become Mr. Olympia by accident. They bought in, and they went after the goal with dedication. If you want to have balance and you are comfortable being average, that is completely fine with me. I do not condemn it. My audience is people who want more, people who want to dive deep and achieve something worth talking about, and it is for you that I am writing right now.

If you want this, you must develop the mindset that you are going to commit to the goal and follow through no matter what. There is no other way. Anyone who tries to sell you the easy way is scamming you. At the end of the day, you are either in or you are out. It is binary. If you settle for something less than full commitment, you will never see your best realized. The Scripture says be either hot or cold, because lukewarm is spit out. There ain't no such things as halfway crooks.

Chapter 15: No Discipline Is Pleasant At The Time

[11] No discipline seems pleasant at the time, but painful. Later on, however, it produces a harvest of righteousness and peace for those who have been trained by it.

Hebrews 12:11 (NIV)

I actually learned this Scripture while listening to the Dave Ramsey radio show while food shopping one day. I am a big fan of Dave because he espouses, in the world of finance, the same principles I advocate in the world of fitness. While his show is very entertaining, you don't need to listen for more than an hour to understand his system for helping people achieve financial independence. His strategy is to get out of debt, establish a fund for emergency, and then when you don't owe anyone money in payments, to take that money and invest it, and rinse and repeat until you achieve your target wealth. He has a clear structure that anyone can understand. But, he gets caller after caller in the same mess of debt which far exceeds income. When he drills down, more often than not the caller has usually failed not for lack of understanding, but because they were impulsive and their dedication waivered when tempted, which caused them to incur more debt. The root issue is an inability to understand the principle of delayed gratification. The same is true with lifting.

The principle of delayed gratification is the ability of an individual to delay an award, or something that feels good in the here and now, for a later award, which far surpasses the immediate award. The trouble is that when we begin a training and nutrition regimen, we don't see the results right away, the body takes time to adapt. Training and nutrition require consistency to be effective. When that happens, it can be easy to doubt. When you don't see the muscle right away, you can be inclined to skip workouts, or even to quit. It could be that your squat is not quite right and takes some time to get off the ground. If you don't see the fat loss right away, it can be difficult to deprive yourself of the things you used to eat. Most people who quit will quit at the beginning, because it can be hard for some people to visualize the goal and consider that goal a reality.

This is where the concepts we have been previously discussing come to life. You must believe in your system, and you must have the discipline to follow through on it. This means continuing to show up for your squat workout until you get it right, or continuing to train before you have seen the muscle gain or fat loss manifest. I remember when I first started training in the way I have described in this book. I would wear an extra-large shirt every day and say to myself I am going to train until I can fill out this shirt. When you have discipline, you continue to show up. You keep the goal in your mind, and don't let anything else in. Henry Ford once said "obstacles are those frightful things you see when you take your eyes off your goal." Focus on the physique you want, focus on the bench press/squat/deadlift you want, focus on whatever your end goal is, and don't let anything else in.

Any true discipline, many times, will not be pleasant while being performed. It's difficult to pull the trigger and make a full commitment to this. It's difficult to deprive yourself of the temporal pleasures you used to enjoy, be it junk food or staying out drinking with your friends. It's difficult when the alarm goes off at 4 a.m., when you had just gotten home from work at 10 p.m., or you have to train late at night or in the middle of the night. It's difficult when you get nauseous just walking into the gym thinking about the deadlift workout you are about to do. I get it, I've been there. But that's only half the story. The deprivation of the temporal pleasures leads to a gratification that is much better than any of the short-term pleasures combined.

I guarantee you that the joy you will feel when you reach your goal will make all of the sacrifices worth it. The joy you will feel when you hit that first 315 squat, 405 squat, 495 squat when you could barely do 185 to start will be tremendous. It will be a tremendous feeling when at the end of the year you hit that first 315 bench, when at the beginning of the year you could only hit 225. It's like an Olympic athlete, every day of his or her entire life is spent working toward the event they compete in, all for one moment in the Olympic games. And to get to the Olympics to win, even to be in the Olympics with the chance to win, is worth every sacrifice they ever made, and more. Even as a viewer, I am captivated by the Olympics because when an athlete stands on the podium with their flag raised, I can feel their emotion, I can feel the culmination of the pain, the struggle, and the sacrifice. But because they executed, because they did what others would not, they got to stand in a place where the common man will never stand. They got their moment on the podium. It wasn't done for money, it wasn't done for fame, it was done because it's what they love and many times just to prove to themselves that they could go the distance and see their goals realized. While the discipline required to get to that point was not easy or pleasant, where they got as a result far exceeded any temporal pleasure they could have indulged in.

Now, be warned, when you make the commitment I am describing, the average people around you will scorn you and say manipulative things like "you don't have a life" or "don't you want to have a life?" You, being adamantine strong, will be able to confidently turn to them and say "what I am doing *is* life, in its purest and highest sense." What does the average person mean when they say "don't you want to have a life?" Is "life" to them performing a series of meaningless tasks for surface and temporal enjoyment, while enduring their work as a necessary evil? We who are adamantine strong know that the "life" we seek is directly linked to the work that we do, and the advancement and achievement we seek. "Life" to us is hitting that new PR, becoming the best we can be, accumulating each day, like money in a bank account, toward a goal for which we have passion and love. "Life" to us is the pursuit, the hunt. The advancement and growth is the key to fulfillment; true, long-lasting fulfillment. The difference between the weak individual and the adamantine strong individual is a mindset, a vision of what is possible.

To me, at least, "life" is being able to look back at my first meet where I squatted 352, and to look at my last meet, three years later, where I squatted 500, and to the future, wherein I plan to squat 525. Life to me is the feeling when there is 100%+ on the deadlift bar, and the judge says the bar is loaded. Life to me is waking up with ambition and purpose, and not with fear and apathy. Life to me is the knowledge that by the grace of God I am in a position to go out and accomplish anything I set my mind to. Life to me is that when I am old and dying, I can be at full peace knowing that I held nothing back, left nothing on the table. So when someone tells you that "you don't have a life," just smile with the wisdom and knowledge that it is that person who knows nothing about "life," and what that word really means.

For us, it's the joy of progress, the honor of commitment, the pride that comes from performing well and being strong, and the principles it takes to get there. We don't live like the common person because we want to be more than a common person, we want to do something that makes us proud of ourselves and brings us joy. I promise you, if you make this commitment, and really follow through, you will reach a more complete joy and fullness that could never have been reached by giving in to short-term indulgences. When you dig further, you will realize that this same logic can then be applied to everything in your life, and then you will know the truth, and the truth will set you free.

Chapter 16: Adamantine Strong

What I hope you all have gotten from this book is that there is no mystery to any of this. Your success does not come down to not having access to some magic supplement or drug, it does not come down to your genetics, and it does not come down to you being less than someone else for some reason. What I hope you have seen, and what I hope we have arrived at, is a set of principles, or guideposts. We have discussed the principle of building a logical structure, not just doing random things. We talked about the difference between training and exercise. As Denzel Washington once said at a commencement speech, don't confuse movement with progress. If you are doing some sort of program/class/system and you cannot quantify your progress from year to year, it's garbage. We who aspire to be adamantine strong will not settle for anything less than quantifiable growth. This does not mean there will not be setbacks on bumps in the road, it just means that you set your path to increase, not to go in a circle.

We have also talked about the importance of perseverance. If you are tough enough to hang around even after things get tough, when the beginner's gains are gone and you have to fight for every single inch, you will see what I mean. There are times when you may feel frustrated, times when you may feel lost, times when you think you are going to break that PR and then don't. Everyone who has done this at a high level has experienced this. No matter what, you keep moving forward and you keep putting your best foot forward, and eventually the ice will break. Thomas Edison once said that "many of life's failures are people who did not realize how close they were to success when they gave up." Don't give up. Keep going.

We also talked about seeing the goal in your mind. Seeing yourself with the physique that you want, seeing yourself hit that deadlift you want to hit. Hebrews 11 says "faith is the substance of things hoped for, the evidence of things not seen." You must believe that your vision is real. If you don't believe that your dream is real, you will be more likely to quit on it. And if you don't believe in your own dream, then no one else will either. You must be an active force in the world. Anything of true value demands the payment upfront; this includes education, business, lifting, relationships, so on and so forth. Phil Heath trains the entire year for one day, the Mr. Olympia contest, and he only sees the finished product on that day. You have to be willing to pay the price to see the reward.

We talked about not making excuses, and as a byproduct, not being delusional. Anyone can make an excuse for not doing anything, it's easy, and that's why most people do it. It is hard to analyze yourself objectively. It is hard to admit your failure is your fault. However, when you do this, it paves the way for tremendous growth. You are not a victim, you are a conqueror. Your circumstances may be worse compared to some other people, but that does not provide you with an excuse for not getting the job done. It's up to you to be better, it's up to you to be tougher. Don't worry about other people, just execute.

At the end of the day, what this all comes down to is understanding these basic principles, which I have tried my best to explain to you, and applying them every single day throughout your training career. I want you to come out of this feeling empowered, focused, and ready to tackle this challenge. I want you to choose to be different. I want you to commit to your goal and your vision, and I want to see you succeed. I want you to be the hero of your own story. I don't want you to fall into the trap of normalcy, of compromise, of mediocrity. I want you to hold yourself to a high standard, to value yourself, to love yourself.

In this book, you have been exposed to the tools that you will need to organize your training and to progress. The next is to continue studying and learning. You now have a framework by which to file everything you read and every program you see. You will be able to tell whether it's a beginner program, and intermediate program, and advanced program, or just garbage. From there, fearlessness, take what you know and apply it, do it, challenge yourself. As you progress and you begin to learn more, impart your wisdom on others. You will learn as much from them as they do from you. Eventually, you will achieve control, mastery. You will be able to use any device in the gym to work toward your goal. You will manipulate exercises and techniques to reach the adaptation that you want.

I suspect that once you apply these principles, you will be hooked. You will not be worried about the things you used to be worried about. You will change. You will be focused. You will be tougher. You will be compassionate (because you know what it took to get there). You will be grateful. You will be more at peace. You will be happier. You will be a better spouse, a better parent, a better son or daughter. You will be proud. You will be someone people look up to. You will be adamantine strong.

Special Thank You

The author would like to extend a special thank you to Strong & Shapely Gym in East Rutherford, New Jersey, for providing a venue for the pictures. A further thank you to Victory Photographs for taking the high-quality demonstration pictures that appear on the cover and in text. I would also like to thank my wife and family for their love and support. Without them, this would not have been possible.